Yaokun Zhang

OPTICAL COHERENCE TOMOGRAPHY GUIDED LASER-COCHLEOSTOMY

Optical Coherence Tomography guided Laser-Cochleostomy

by

Yaokun Zhang

KIT Scientific Publishing

Dissertation, Karlsruher Institut für Technologie (KIT)
Fakultät für Informatik, 2014

Tag der mündlichen Prüfung: 7. Februar 2014
Referenten: Prof. Dr.-Ing. Heinz Wörn
Prof. Dr. med. Dr. h.c. Thomas Klenzner

Impressum

KIT Scientific Publishing

Karlsruher Institut für Technologie (KIT)
KIT Scientific Publishing
Straße am Forum 2
D-76131 Karlsruhe

KIT Scientific Publishing is a registered trademark of Karlsruhe Institute of Technology. Reprint using the book cover is not allowed.

www.ksp.kit.edu

Print on Demand 2015

ISBN 978-3-7315-0302-6
DOI 10.5445/KSP/1000044633

Optical Coherence Tomography guided Laser-Cochleostomy

zur Erlangung des akademischen Grades eines

Doktors der Ingenieurwissenschaften

von der Fakultät für Informatik
des Karlsruher Instituts für Technologie (KIT)

genehmigte

Dissertation

von

Yaokun Zhang

aus Shanghai

Tag der mündlichen Prüfung:	07. February 2014
Erster Gutachter:	Prof. Dr.-Ing. Heinz Wörn
Zweiter Gutachter:	Prof. Dr. med. Dr. h.c. Thomas Klenzner

给我亲爱的老爸老妈和征征

Abstract

In this work, an optical coherence tomography (OCT) guided laser-cochleostomy system has been proposed and successfully realized for future surgical applications at the inner ear. After appropriate image quality enhancement of the intraoperatively acquired OCT scans, the position of the bone-endosteum-perilymph boundary can be detected several hundred micrometers before its exposure to the air. Position and duration of the succeeding ablation pulses are planned based on the residual bone thickness above the critical structure. OCT itself is also used as a highly accurate optical tracking system for motion compensation between the target area and the laser optics. During *ex vivo* experimental evaluation on fresh porcine cochleae, the ablation process terminated automatically when the thickness of the residual tissue layer uniformly reached a predefined value. The shape of the resulting channel bottom converged to the natural curvature of the endosteal layer without injuring the critical structure. Preliminary measurements in OCT scans indicated that the mean absolute accuracy of the shape approximation was only around $20\mu m$. A closed-loop control of the endosteum preserving laser-cochleostomy with the accuracy on tens of micrometer scale is thereby established.

Acknowledgement

This doctoral thesis was accomplished during my work as researcher in the Medical Group (MeGI) at the Institute for Process Control and Robotics (IPR) of the Karlsruhe Institute of Technology (KIT). This work was funded by the German Research Foundation (DFG) within the scope of the project OCT-LABS.

First of all, I would like to thank every one who contributed to the success of the project and the writing of this thesis. I also greatly appreciate the help of my friends, colleagues and fellow classmates during the whole period of my education and my life.

I would like to extend my sincere gratitude to Professor Heinz Wörn, my supervisor and the head of IPR, for his mentorship and guidance during my PhD study. Working at the IPR was the most important step for my academic and career development. I am also greatly indebted to my second supervisor and project partner, Professor Thomas Klenzner. The valuable discussion with him and his instructions have helped me a lot during the collaboration. I would like to gratefully and sincerely thank my group leader Dr. Jörg Raczkowsky for his mentorship, understanding, friendship and trust. The eight-year working experience in his group has become the cornerstone of my long-term career goals.

Without the collaboration with my project partners, Professor Robert Huber, Wolfgang Wieser and Marcel Weller, I would never be able to finish my thesis. I also appreciate the contribution of my students Mark Brenner, Dirk Gutting, Shen Hu, Yicheng Liu, Johannes Meyer and Bo Zhang. Special thanks go to my colleague Tom Pfeiffer and assistant Ruomin Sun for the days and nights we worked together in the lab during the most crucial time of the project.

I am very grateful for the friendship of the MeGI group members: Tim Beyl, Thorsten Brenneck, Julien Mintenbeck, Philip Nicolai and Luzie Schreiter. Beside the daily work at the institute, they also helped me a lot as a foreigner to overcome many intercultural problems in everyday life. I also owe my sincere gratitude to my friends Qi Chen, Wenjie Yan and Ting Yu for their inspiring advices and discussion regarding my thesis. In particular, I would like to express my special appreciation to Mirko Kunze and Chengchao Qu who have in addition spent a lot of time reading and correcting my manuscript.

Finally, I would like to thank my parents and my wife for their unending love, patience and support over the years. They gave me the courage to overcome any difficulties that I confronted.

THANK YOU ALL!

Yaokun Zhang

Contents

CHAPTER 1
Introduction

Motivation Cochleostomy is a vital step of cochlear implantation (figure 1.1). Its purpose is to create an artificial insertion channel in the bony shell of the cochlea, through which the soft electrode array of the implant can be inserted into the scala tympani and stimulate the auditory nerves.

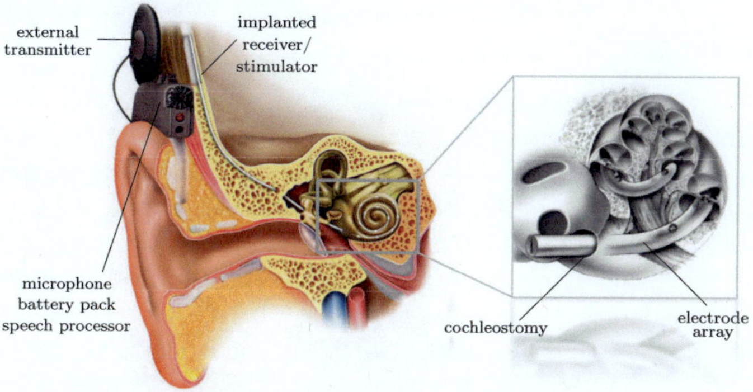

Figure 1.1: Illustration of a cochleostomy [MED09], which is an artificial corridor on the bony cochlea for inserting the electrode array into the scala tympani.

The inner side of the scala tympani is covered by a thin lining membrane (endosteum) protecting the chamber filled with fluid perilymph. During the process of cochleostomy, injury to this critical structure must be avoided while a defined removal of the overlying bone tissue is required, so that the leakage of the perilymph before the electrode array insertion can be prevented and the risk of infection can be reduced.

Conventionally, the cochleostomy is drilled manually by the surgeon with diamond burrs and the reachable precision is mainly dependent on the skills and experiences of the surgeon. Due to the small size of the cochleostomy (<1 mm in diameter) and the low thickness of the fragile endosteum (<50 μm), the required accuracy almost reaches the limit of the human capabilities and results in extremely high demands on the surgeon. A computer aided micro-surgery system is therefore desired to support the surgeons.

Researches throughout the last decade have revealed that short-pulsed infrared lasers such as Er:YAG (wavelength 2.9 μm) or CO_2 (wavelength 9.6 μm and 10.6 μm) lasers are suitable for the ablation of bone tissue. Compared with the conventional surgical instruments, the laser ablation allows contactless removal of bone tissue in the absence of any mechanical stress to the delicate structures, providing more safety to the patient. Moreover, the tiny tissue volume ablated by each single pulse enables an accurate control of the ablation depth, so that the natural shape of the cochlear endosteum can be approached more precisely. However, a main question remains unsolved: how to detect the actual position of the membrane during the ablation process and how to arrange the laser pulses accordingly?

Being able to provide tomographic images of the target tissue with an axial resolution on micrometre scale, optical coherence tomography (OCT) is a promising candidate for monitoring the bottom of the ablated channel during the process of cochleostomy. The combination of these two technologies may result in a closed-loop control of the laser-bone ablation during the cochleostomy, namely *OCT guided laser-cochleostomy*, which may provide a solution to the defined hard tissue removal with simultaneous protection of the critical cochlear endosteum underneath.

Scientific Challenges Although both OCT and laser ablation systems are nowadays widely used in the medical field and industry, their typical applications are separated and independent of each other. A bridge connecting these two cutting-edge technologies does not exist yet. Therefore, the main scientific challenge of this doctoral thesis is: how to realise the closed-loop control of laser-bone ablation under the monitoring with OCT?

In order to achieve this goal, the following five questions have to be answered within the scope of this doctoral thesis:

i. While monitoring the process of laser-cochleostomy, what kinds of distortions and noises does OCT suffer from? How can they be corrected and suppressed?

ii. How to detect the position of the cochlear endosteum in OCT scans and how to measure the thickness of the residual bone tissue above it?

iii. Where should the laser pulses on the next layer be applied and how to choose the best pulse duration?

iv. How to integrate and coordinate the OCT and the ablating laser?

v. What accuracy can be reached by OCT guided laser ablation?

Outline In this work, a closed-loop control for OCT guided laser-cochleostomy will be conceived and developed step by step. In chapter 2, the background of cochlear implantation and fundamentals of the laser-bone ablation are introduced. A comparison between candidate sensor methodologies for the closed-loop control of the laser ablation is made afterwards. Chapter 3 gives an introduction of the working principle of OCT. Feasibility studies of using OCT as an online imaging system for the detection of the cochlear endosteum are reported and the control loop of the laser-cochleostomy is proposed. Basic image processing and mature image segmentation techniques, which play an important role in analysing the OCT images acquired during the laser ablation, are summarised in chapter 4.

The following two chapters focus on establishing the desired control loop. The scientific challenges i-iii are answered in chapter 5. By means of analysing the properties of the OCT images in detail, methods for correcting the artefacts in the scans and enhancing image quality are developed. The refractive index of bone tissue is measured directly in the OCT images. A novel speckle noise reduction technique, *history compounding* is invented. The online detection of the endosteum position is then realised and an ablation strategy regarding the measured three-dimensional residual bone thickness profile above the endosteum is designed. The OCT and CO_2 laser systems are connected in chapter 6, giving answers to the questions iv and v. After physically combining both systems, the mapping between both coordinate systems is precisely determined. The OCT itself is innovatively utilized as an optical tracking system to compensate tiny movements of the patient. The proposed closed-loop control of the laser-cochleostomy is thereby established and experimentally evaluated afterwards.

The complete workflow of OCT guided laser-cochleostomy is summarised in chapter 7 and the doctoral thesis closes with an outlook on further research issues.

CHAPTER 2 Laser-Cochleostomy

In this chapter, background knowledges about laser-cochleostomy will be presented. Starting with the anatomy of the cochlea, the cochlear implantation and the conventional cochleostomy are briefly introduced and the difficulties of the process are analysed. The concept of laser-cochleostomy is conceived and an introduction to the mechanism of laser bone ablation is given, followed by a summary of preliminary works of performing cochleostomy with a short-pulsed CO_2 laser at own institute. Finally, an overview of candidate sensor technologies for controlling the endosteum preserving laser-cochleostomy is made and the most feasible choice is decided.

2.1 Cochleostomy

2.1.1 Cochlea

Cochlea is a spiral shaped structure in the inner ear (compare figure 1.1 and figure 2.1a), which is responsible for transforming mechanical vibrations captured by the tympanic membrane into nerve impulses. The outer shell of the cochlea consists of compact bone[1] and protects the coiled cochlear canal which contains three fluid filled (explained below)

[1] There are two kinds of bone tissue: compact bone (also called cortical bone) and cancellous bone. Compact bone is much denser, harder and stiffer than the other one, whose main function is to support the body and protect organs, more details refer to [BLW87].

chambers: scala vestibuli, scala media and scala tympani, as illustrated in figure 2.1a-b. The inner side of the bony shell is covered by a thin layer of lining membrane (endosteum), which is exactly the critical structure to be protected during the cochleostomy (see also section 2.1.2). The Reissner's membrane divides the scala vestibuli and scala media apart while the scala media and scala tympani are separated by basilar membrane. The organ of Corti is a matrix of cells on the top of the basilar membrane, to which the sensory hair cells are attached.

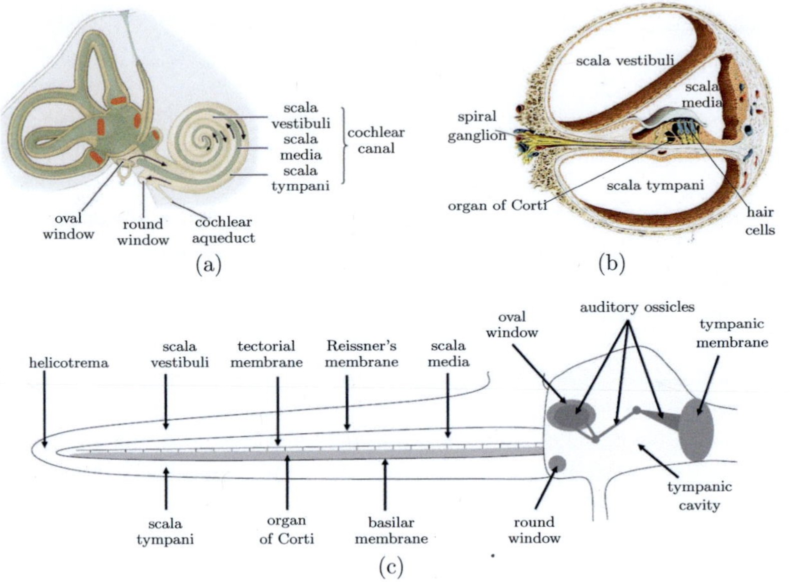

Figure 2.1: Anatomy of cochlea: (a) schematic diagram of the cochlea and (b) the cross section of the cochlear canal [GSV12]; (c) illustration of uncoiled cochlea and middle ear [Kah09].

The scala vestibuli and scala tympani are filled with perilymph and the fluid in the scala media is endolymph. The first two scalae merge with each other at the apex of the cochlear canal through the helicotrema (at the tip of uncoiled cochlea in figure 2.1c). The vibration of the tympanic membrane is mechanically transmitted by the auditory ossicles (three small bones in of the middle ear) and coupled into the scala vestibuli through the oval window, resulting in back and forth movement of the perilymph inside the scala vesitibuli and scala tympani along the arrow marked path in the sub-figure a.

The scala tympani terminates at the round window covered by the round window membrane, which is deformed passively by the pressure of the perilymph in the opposite direction of the oval window movement, allowing the fluid to move in the scalae. The oscillations of the perilymph in turn initiate a travelling wave of displacement along the basilar membrane. This motion is sensed by the hair cells in the organ of Corti, which amplify and transform the vibration into nerve impulses and then transmitted to the brain via the auditory nerves. Detailed description of the physiology of cochlea can be found in [PAF+01, JSS01, WD08].

2.1.2 Cochlear Implant and Cochleostomy

Cochlear Implant For the patients with severe hearing loss due to damage to or complete destruction of the sensory hair cells whose auditory nerves are still functional, cochlea implant provides the possibility to bypass the hair cells by directly stimulating the surviving neurons in the auditory nerve [WD08], so that the hearing ability of the patient could be partially restored.

In general, a cochlear implant consists of two main parts: external and implanted parts (illustration see figure 1.1). The external part includes microphone, speech processor, battery and transmitter, which are responsible for sensing sound in the environment and transforming the signal to stimuli for the implanted electrodes. The power and stimulus information is transmitted by the external transmitter across the skin into the implanted receiver. The receiver decodes and generates stimuli according to the received instructions. The stimulation of the auditory nerve is then produced by currents delivered through an intracochlear electrode array carrying up to 22 electrodes placed in the scala tympani [Leu05, MED09, Nip09].

Cochleostomy There are two possibilities to insert the electrode array into the scala tympani, either through the round window or through an artificial opening drilled on the bony shell of the cochlea, the so called *cochleostomy*. Due to the anatomical structure of the cochlea, the orientation of the round window may not always be convenient for the insertion and risks to damage the basilar membrane [ZB85, Kah09]. Takahashi et al. [THST95] stated that about 30-50% of the patients receiving cochlear implant encounter pathological closure of round window, which makes it difficult to perform the insertion through the round window. In such cases, the cochleostomy can provide a "straighter" insertion path [WD08], so that the difficulty and risk of the insertion can be reduced correspondingly (see also the example shown in figure 1.1, where the electrode array has to be bent upwards if inserted through the round window). Consequently, cochleostomy is nowadays widely applied for the cochlear implantation surgery [BTSR05, AB07, ARG+07, KKS+09, BAB10].

In general, a small number of hair cells may remain for some patients, usually in the apical (low frequency) part of the cochlea [WD08]. These patients may still have some level of existing residual hearing. Unable to preserve this residual hearing, the intracochlear implant was only recommended for completely deaf ears during the early years, until the *soft surgery technique* was proposed by Lehnhardt [Leh93], which consists of a small, localized cochleostomy and a gentle electrode insertion.

The cochleostomy using this technique is performed in the following procedure: flatten the promontory with a large burr; create the cochleostomy with a smaller burr and expose endosteum of scala tympani; smooth the bony edges and generate limited opening of the scala tympani that matches the size of the electrode array [RRL95, Coh97, JAB+05], as illustrated in figure 2.2. A key point during this procedure is to reserve the endosteum enclosing the perilymph until immediately before the electrode array insertion to avoid the loss of the fluid.

Although operated with great care, the burr frequently tears or perforates the endosteum of the scala tympani despite the surgeon's best efforts [RW06]. A major difficulty of the cochleostomy is its small diameter (less than 1 mm) and the tiny thickness of the fragile endosteum. As a result, the required accuracy is so high that almost exceeds the limit of the human capabilities.

Meanwhile, the cochleostomy is performed under OP-microscope and the surgeons visually recognize the exposure of the endosteum by its color that is lighter than the surrounding bone tissue [JAB+05, Kah09]. However, the drill bit itself blocks the visual contact of the surgeon to the channel bottom while deepening the channel (figure 2.2b), so that the drilling and visual monitoring have to be performed in turn but not simultaneously. The surgeons have to rely on the haptic feedback from the burr and feel the stiffness of the channel bottom while the view is blocked, making the task risky and demanding.

Moreover, an inherent shortcoming of mechanical drilling is that the resulting channel bottom has the same shape as the burr that is convex in the direction of the drilling (figure 2.2b). But, the natural shape of the cochlea is convex towards outside (figure 2.1a-b, see also figure 3.6-3.8), i.e. in the opposite direction of the drilling. As a result, while the drill bit already touches the endosteum in the middle part of the channel, some residual bone tissue still remains near the wall of the cochleostomy (figure 2.2b). In such a case, it is a challenging task to expose a sufficiently large area of the endosteum that matches the diameter of the implant without damaging the already exposed thin membrane in the middle. A widening and smoothing step illustrated in figure 2.2c has to be performed, which further increases the difficulty and risk of the procedure. Consequently, performing the cochleostomy requires very high skills and experiences of the surgeon.

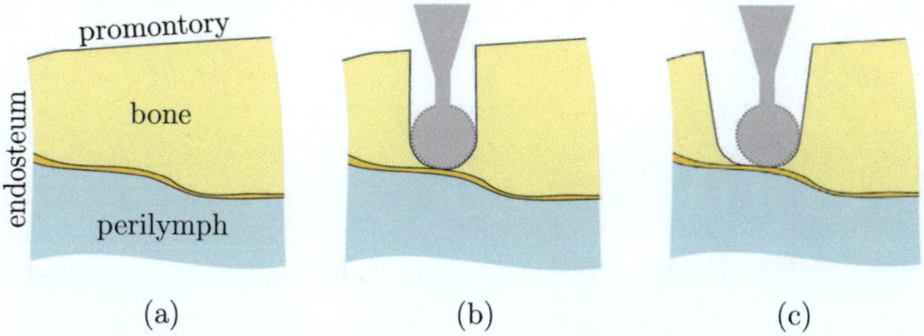

Figure 2.2: Drilling process of a cochleostomy: (a) flattening of the promontory; (b) exposing the endosteum of the scala tympani with a small burr (ϕ =0.6 mm); (c) smoothing the bony edges and creating a limited opening that matches the diameter of the electrode array [Kah09].

In addition to the difficulties stated above, the drilling process of the cochleostomy is also associated with significant acoustic trauma and potentially allows bone dust to enter scala tympani [RW06]. High frequency vibration of the fragile cochlea is also unavoidable during the drilling process, which might further injure the structure.

Mechatronic-assisted Cochleostomy A mechatronic-assisted microsurgery system might provide a solution to support the surgeons to ensure a reproducible precision during this highly demanding surgery. For this purpose, robotic systems are common choices, either using a highly precise hexapod [Nga06, KNK+09] (figure 2.3a)or a standard robot arm [MRB+09, EBO+09]. Based on preoperative planning in CT scans, the robot is navigated to perform the drilling without violating critical structures like the facial nerve and the chorda tympani until reaching the stop point located on the endosteum. Unfortunately, the accuracy of the stop point in the planning data is limited by the resolution of the CT scan, which is about 0.1-0.25 mm in clinical routine and insufficient regarding the thickness of the endosteum that is only several tens micros. Unavoidable intraoperative registration and navigation errors further worsen the situation.

The workgroup of Brett et al. [BDZA$^+$14, DAJ$^+$13] therefore developed autonomous surgical robotic systems with real time haptic feedback. The critical structure is discriminated by analyzing the force and torque measured from the tip of the drill bit (figure 2.3b). The drilling will be ceased when a significant change in force and torque occurs, indicating that the endosteum is reached.

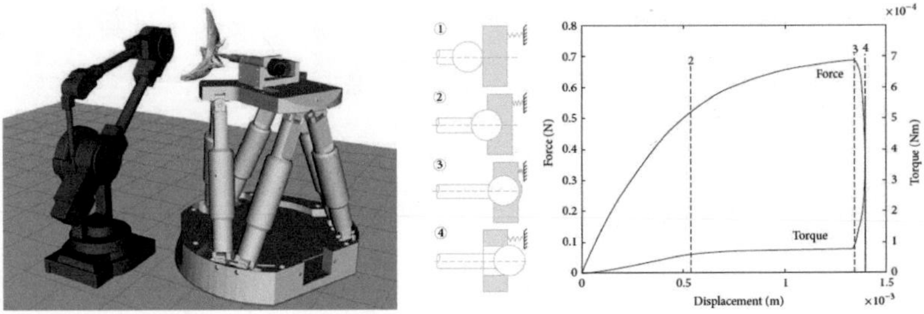

(a) (b)

Figure 2.3: (a) A typical mechatronic-assisted microsurgery setup [Nga06], where the drill is attached to a highly accurate hexapod. (b) The simulated force and torque feedback from the drill bit at different stage of the process [TDP$^+$10].

However, these solutions still use conventional drilling tools and are therefore not able to overcome the inherent shortcomings of the mechanical drilling such as limited channel shape, acoustic trauma, bone dust, vibration etc.

Laser-Cochleostomy: Conception In order to overcome the difficulties of the conventional cochleostomy and to reduce the trauma of the patient, Kahrs et al. [Kah09] have developed a laser-cochleostomy system (details will be introduced in section 2.3.1), which uses a short-pulsed CO_2 laser instead of the burr to perform the drilling.

Compared to the mechanical drilling process described above, the removal of bone tissue with laser, known as *laser-bone ablation*, provides the following advantages:

- Precise control of the channel shape:
  Each single laser pulse ablates a tiny tissue volume that is circa $200\,\mu\text{m}$ in diameter and 5-150 μm in depth. A flexible channel bottom geometry can be achieved by applying the pulses to appropriate positions, so that the endosteum can be approached more precisely without injury to it (figure 2.4).
- Contactless ablation (see also figure 2.8):
  No mechanical stress will be applied to the fragile cochlea, preventing injury due to vibration. The visual contact to the channel bottom will not be blocked, either.
- Lower ablation noises:
  The ablation induced acoustic emission is much lower than mechanical drilling and brings less acoustic trauma accordingly.
- Less bone dust:
  Most irradiated tissues are evaporated and the rest part is also brought away by the ablation induced micro-explosion (detail see section 2.2.2) immediately, so that almost no bone dust will remain in the cochleostomy.

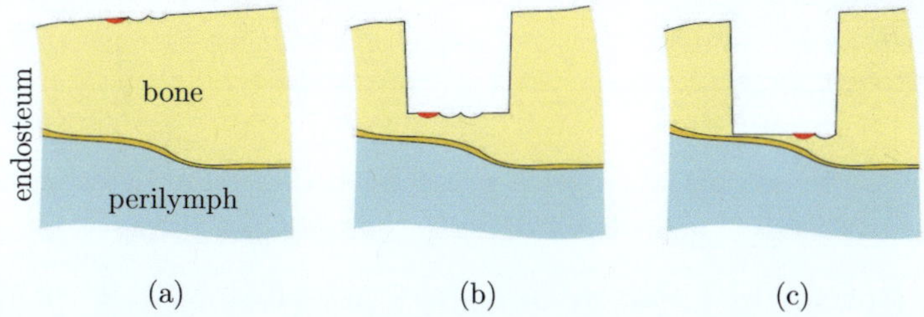

Figure 2.4: The concept of laser-cochleostomy: the bony shell of the cochlea is ablated pulse by pulse using a short-pulsed CO_2 laser and the shape of the endosteum can be approached more precisely. The red spots denote the currently being ablated tiny tissue volume [Kah09].

Consequently, the laser ablation provides almost an ideal solution to the problems of conventional cochleostomy. In the next section, its mechanism will be introduced in detail.

2.2 Laser-Bone Ablation

2.2.1 Basic Knowledges

Laser The word "laser" is an acronym for *light amplification by stimulated emission of radiation.* The main component of a laser device is the optical resonator containing an active medium shown in figure 2.5a. As its name suggests, laser is generated by the stimulated emission of atoms in the active medium. Usually, the electrons of an atom occupy the position with the lowest possible energy and the atom with the electrons in this configuration is at *ground state.* While photons with enough energy hit an atom, lead one or more electrons of the atom to be excited to the orbits with higher energy level, the atom is then at *excited state.* Suppose the numbers of atoms at ground and excited states are N_1 and N_2 respectively. Then it is required to satisfy $N_2 > N_1$ in order to make laser operation possible, known as *population inversion.* Population inversion is realised by pumping up the atoms to excited state with the energy level that is two or three levels higher than the ground state using an external pumping source.

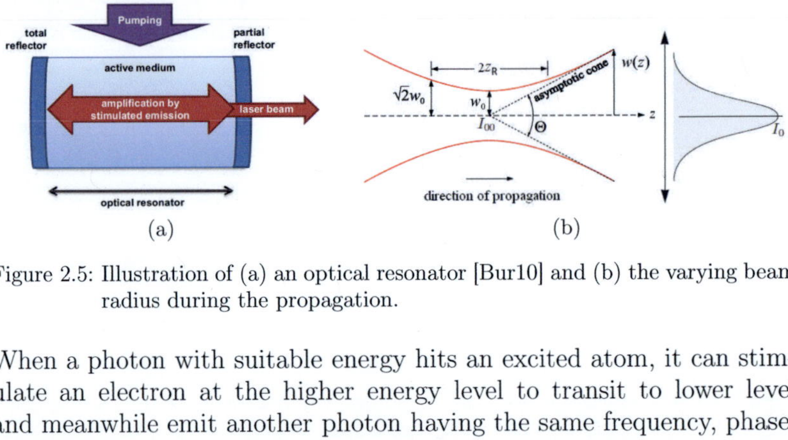

(a) (b)

Figure 2.5: Illustration of (a) an optical resonator [Bur10] and (b) the varying beam radius during the propagation.

When a photon with suitable energy hits an excited atom, it can stimulate an electron at the higher energy level to transit to lower level and meanwhile emit another photon having the same frequency, phase, polarisation and propagation direction as the incident one. Such a phenomenon is exactly the so called *stimulated emission.* The incident photon and newly emitted photon are reflected between the two reflectors of the resonator back and forth, resulting in more and more photons released by stimulated emission and the intensity of the beam is thus amplified, until its intensity is high enough to penetrate the partial reflector and emitted outwards. Due to the same properties of the photons, a laser beam is monochromatic, coherent and unidirectional.

Gaussian Beam After leaving the resonator, the laser light can be classified by its *Transverse Electro Magnetic* (TEM) mode, describing the electromagnetic field pattern of radiation measured in a plane perpendicular to the propagation direction of the beam. Particularly, the CO_2 laser and OCT (see chapter 3) used in this thesis have the TEM_{00} mode, whose intensity distributions can be described as

$$I(r,z) = I_{00}\left(\frac{w_0}{w(z)}\right)^2 \exp\left(-\frac{2r^2}{w^2(z)}\right) \tag{2.1}$$

where z denotes the position on the optical axis; r is the radial distance to the optical axis; I_{00} is the intensity at the centre of the beam at its waist (explained below); w_0 and $w(z)$ are the beam radii at the beam waist as well as any given axial position z respectively. Equation (2.1) is a Gaussian functions and the TEM_{00} mode is hence named as *Gaussian beam*. Figure 2.5b illustrates this distribution.

It can further be observed that instead of being perfectly collimated, the beam radius varies during propagation and reaches a minimum value w_0 at one particular position, known as the *beam waist*. For a beam with the wavelength λ, the variation of the beam radius can be described by the following equation:

$$w(z) = w_0\sqrt{1+\left(\frac{\lambda z}{\pi w_0^2}\right)^2} \tag{2.2}$$

It indicates that Gaussian beams do not diverge linearly: near the beam waist, the divergence angle is extremely small; far from the waist, the beam contours asymptotically approach a so called *asymptotic cone*. The *Rayleigh range* z_{R} is defined at the distance where $w(z) = \sqrt{2}w_0$, denoting the area of the cross section is doubled. Substituting this into equation (2.2), the Rayleigh range is then

$$z_{\text{R}} = \pi w_0^2/\lambda \tag{2.3}$$

The double of the Rayleigh range $2z_{\text{R}}$ defines the *tolerance range* of the beam (marked in 2.5b), within which the beam is considered to be well focused. For laser-material processing (in our case laser-bone ablation) and imaging (in our case OCT-biological tissue imaging), the target surface should always be kept within the Rayleigh range of the beam.

Further details of laser physics can be found in [EE06, PPBS96, Sch07].

Refraction and Reflection While the laser beam propagates along its optical axis z (figure 2.5b) and reaches the target sample surface, or more general, whenever a light reaches the boundary between two different media, part of the incident light will come back to the first medium while the rest part will enter the second medium. These basic phenomena are called *reflection* and *refraction* respectively, as illustrated in figure 2.6, in which the angles θ_i, θ_r and θ_t are the incident angle, reflection angle and refraction angles.

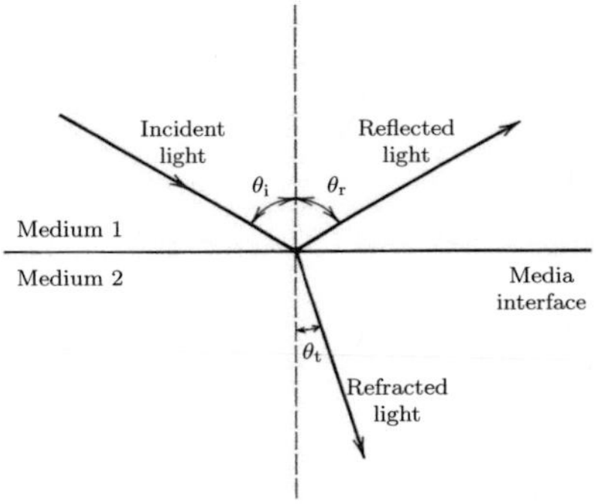

Figure 2.6: Reflection and refraction of light on media interface [YY97].

According to the law of reflection, the reflection angle is always equal to the incident angle. Meanwhile, the refraction angle depends on the velocities of light in the two media. In practice, instead of the velocity of light, the **refractive index** is used more often. The refractive index of a medium is defined by the ratio of the speed of light in vacuum c to that in the material ν as

$$n = c/\nu \tag{2.4}$$

Then, the relation between the incident angle and refraction angle is given by the **Snell's law of refraction**:

$$\frac{\sin\theta_i}{\sin\theta_t} = \frac{n_2}{n_1} \tag{2.5}$$

In particular, if the light is quasi perpendicularly incident, i.e. $\theta_i \approx 0$, and suppose the intensities of the incident, reflected and refracted light are I_i, I_r and I_t respectively, then the fraction of the incident irradiation that is reflected, namely **reflectance**, can be derived from the *Fresnel reflection coefficient* and described by the following equation (detailed derivation refer to [DiM12]):

$$\frac{I_r}{I_i} = \left| \frac{(n_2/n_1) - 1}{(n_2/n_1) + 1} \right|^2 \tag{2.6}$$

The fraction of the refracted part that is transmitted into the second medium can be easily derived by energy conservation accordingly:

$$\frac{I_t}{I_i} = 1 - \frac{I_r}{I_i}$$

2.2.2 Ablation Mechanism

After transmitted into the target tissue, the absorption of the laser radiation plays a major role in the ablation process, which turns the energy of the incident laser beam into heat that initiates the ablation process. The ability of a medium to absorb an electromagnetic radiation can be described by the so called **Lambert-Beer law**:

$$I(z) = I_0 \exp(-\mu z)$$

where z denotes the depth penetrating into the target medium; $I(z)$ is the residual intensity of the laser radiation at z; I_0 is the intensity of the refracted laser beam at the bone surface (i.e. the I_t stated above); μ is the **absorption coefficient** of the medium. The Lambert-Beer law indicates that the intensity of the laser radiation attenuates exponentially due to the absorption. Based on this phenomenon, the **optical penetration depth** z_{opt} is defined as the depth z at which the intensity $I(z)$ has dropped to $1/\mathrm{e}$ (36.8%) of its incident value I_0, yield $z_{opt} = 1/\mu$. It can be further derived that at the position $z = 2/\mu$ and $z = 3/\mu$, the $I(z)$ is dropped to $1/\mathrm{e}^2$ (13.5%) and $1/\mathrm{e}^3$ (5.0%) respectively. The absorption coefficients of typical infrared lasers are very high in bone tissues, as listed in table 2.1, where 2.94 μm is the wavelength of Er:YAG laser and 9.6 μm, 10.6 μm are typical wavelengths of CO_2 lasers.

Table 2.1: Material components (weight proportion) of different kinds of bone tissue and absorption coefficient μ at different infrared wavelengths [Wer06].

μ [cm^{-1}]	weight proportion [%]				wavelength [μm]		
	water	minerals	collagen	lipid	2.94	9.6	10.6
cortical bone	13.5	60	25.5	1	3800	2250	1500
cancellous bone	30.5	34	34	1.5	5900	1300	970
dentin	16.7	67.8	15.5	0	4640	2610	1770
enamel	4.5	95	0.5	0	2170	4470	3080

Taking the CO_2 laser with the wavelength of 10.6 μm as example, the absorption coefficient in compact (cortical) bone tissue is 1500 cm^{-1}. Simple calculation reveals that 63% of the incident laser radiation will be absorbed by the most superficial 6.7 μm tissues and 95% of the energy is deposited within a thin layer of 20 μm.

The fast energy deposition within such a small tissue volume leads to rapid local temperature increase, resulting in melting and evaporation of the irradiated tissue volume. The violent evaporation causes audible micro-explosions, accompanied by material ejection into the air and forming a flame-like ablation plume, as shown in figure 2.7a, leaving a tiny crater with the similar diameter as the laser beam on the tissue surface. Detailed description of this process is available in [VV03, Nie07].

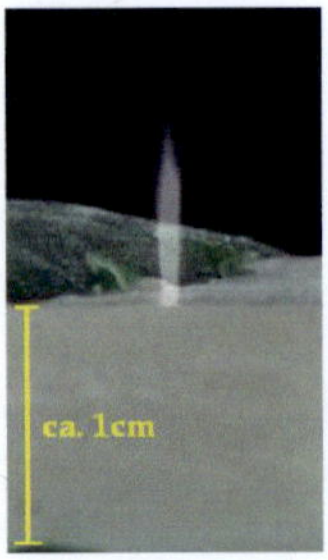

(a)

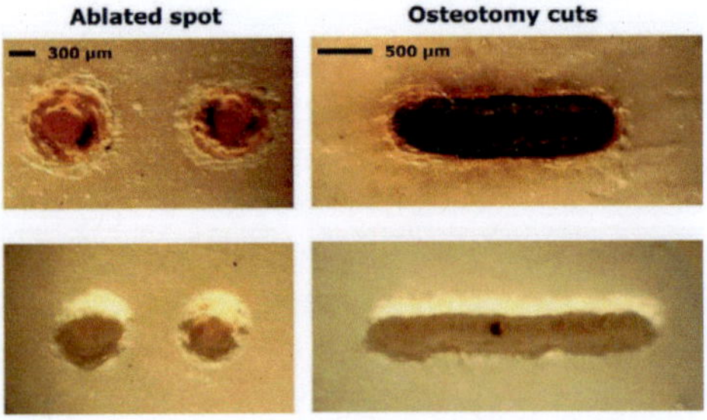

(b)

Figure 2.7: (a) Typical ablation plume during laser ablation on bovine compact bone. (b) Comparison between laser ablation without (above) and with (below) water spray, revealing that water spray can effectively prevent ablation induced thermal injury [KOW08].

However, the high temperature also brings a side effect that the deposited heat is diffused to the surrounding tissue, resulting in severe thermal injury and carbonisation. A simple but effective solution to this problem is to apply cooling water spray to the site of the ablation [IH98, IWA+05, Wer06, KOW08, MMF+08, Bur10], which brings the residual heat away and thus reduce the thermal injury accordingly, as shown in figure 2.7b.

2.2.3 Laser Ablation System Setup

Laser Source In order to perform the conceived laser-cochleostomy, a Rofin Sinar SCx10 CO_2 Laser (Rofin-Sinar Laser GmbH, Hamburg, Germany) is utilized as laser source within the scope of this thesis. It works in TEM_{00} mode and supplies 10.6 μm laser beam with typical pulse duration configurable between 20-100 μs, corresponding to the ablation depth of circa 5-150 μm on compact bone tissue.

Galvanometric Laser Scanner In order to apply the laser pulses precisely and rapidly to the desired positions (see figure 2.4), a laser scanner Colibri 11 (ARGES GmbH, Wackersdorf, Germany) is installed to the laser ablation system. It has two perpendicularly mounted galvanometric scanning mirrors, which can deflect the laser beam in a two-dimensional scan field by changing the mirror angles with an accuracy of $< 20\mu$rad, as shown in figure 2.8.

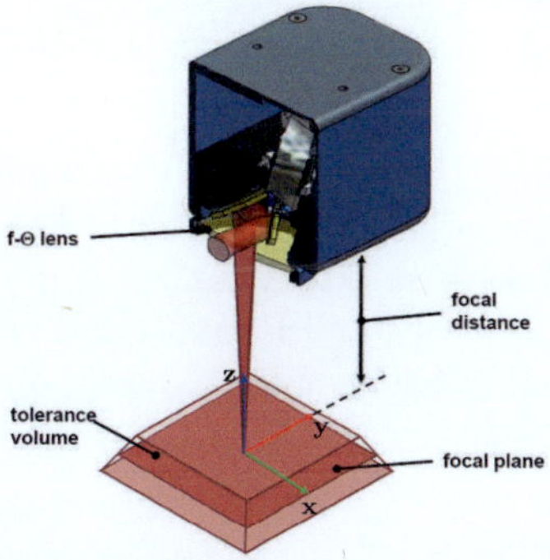

Figure 2.8: Illustration of the ARGES Colibri 11 laser scanner and its working space, adapted from [ARG13, Bur10].

Due to the scanning mechanism, the optical path is inclined while the beam is deflected to the boundary of the scan field, resulting in varying path length during the scanning. The scanner is therefore further equipped with an f-θ lens, which guarantees that the waist of the deflected laser beam is always focused onto a single plane, known as the *focal plane*. As stated in section 2.2.1, the tissue surface to be processed has to be located within the Rayleigh range of the beam. Therefore, the *working space* (also called tolerance volume) of the scanner is a three-dimensional trapezoidal volume centred at the focal plane.

The focused laser spot has the diameter of $200\,\mu$m on the focal plane, which is located at 114 mm from the scanner bottom and has the size of $70 \times 70\,\mathrm{mm}^2$. The thickness of the working space is 4.8 mm.

2.3 Endosteum Preserving Laser-Cochleostomy

2.3.1 Preliminary Works at Own Institute

Robot Assisted Laser Osteotomy Although the circa $70 \times 70 \times 4.8\,\mathrm{mm}^3$ working space is large enough to cover the cochleostomy, it is however challenging to aim the insertion channel with the diameter of only 1 mm from a distance of more than 100 mm. For a precise positioning and orienting of the laser scanner, Burgner et al. [BRW08, BKRW09, BMRW09, Bur10, BMRW10] have developed a robot assisted laser osteotomy system within the scope of the EU-project Accurate Robot Assistant (AccuRobAs).

The system was originally designed to perform general laser osteotomy surgery, i.e. cutting bone tissue with the laser. As a special case of osteotomy, the laser-cochleostomy can also be performed with the system. Pre-operatively, the optimal location and orientation of the laser scanner relative to the patient are planned according to the preoperative CT or MRI (figure 2.9a).

Intra-operatively, the laser scanner is coupled to a robot. After the registration of the patient position, the robot moves the scanner precisely to the planned position with the predefined orientation (figure 2.9b). The ablation procedure conceived in figure 2.4 can be then executed.

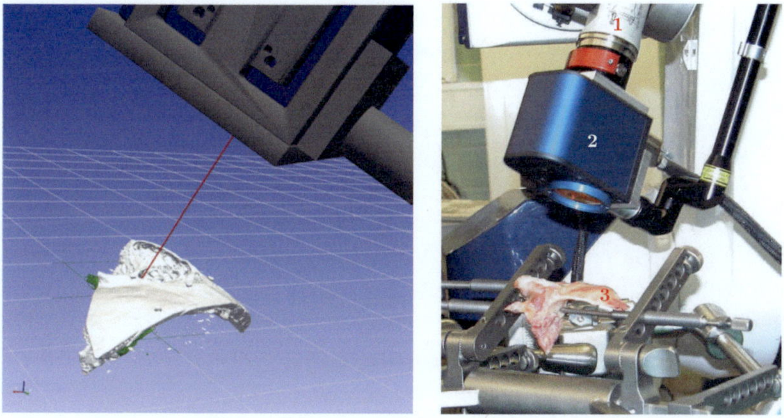

(a) (b)

Figure 2.9: Laser-cochleostomy performed by a robot assisted laser osteotomy system [Bur10]: (a) pre-operative planning; (b) intra-operative execution, where the laser scanner (2) is precisely positioned by a robot (1) to the pre-operatively planned location relative to the patient (3).

However, a key question is: *How to terminate the laser ablation exactly when the underlying critical structure is reached*?

For the robot assisted laser osteotomy system, the control of the ablation process remains open-loop and relies on an empirical model based pre-operative simulation, which determines the number of laser pulses that are needed to achieve the planned channel depth. Due to the complexity of the laser-tissue interaction, a precise modelling of the process is almost impossible so that the simulation cannot provide enough accuracy, which is further limited by individual differences between the patients, the resolution of the CT or MRI imaging ($>1/4$ mm in clinical routine), the unpredictable energy loss in the water spray, etc.

For the desired endosteum preserving laser-cochleostomy, a closed-loop control of the laser ablation is mandatory in order to terminate the ablation process as soon as the critical structure is exposed without applying further pulses onto it.

Visual Control of Laser-Cochleostomy Compared to conventional cochleostomy, the visual contact to the bottom of the insertion channel will not be blocked any more during the laser ablation. Kahrs et al. [KWK+07, KRW+08, Kah09, KBK+10] have taken advantage of this property and developed an online visual control module for the laser-cochleostomy within the scope of the Priority Programme 1124 of the German Research Foundation.

As introduced in section 2.1.2, the surgeon recognizes the exposure of the endosteum by its lighter colour compared with the neighbouring bone tissue. Kahrs et al. have automated this procedure by analysing the images acquired by a video camera attached to the OP-microscope monitoring the cochleostomy (figure 2.10), where the areas of the exposed endosteum is automatically segmented (green area in the figure) and no more pulses are allowed to be applied to these areas.

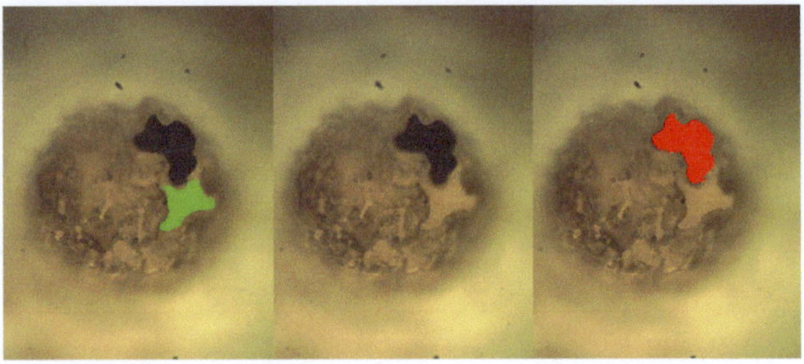

Figure 2.10: Image-based visual control of laser-cochleostomy: automated segmentation of the cochlear endosteum (green) and laser induced membrane perforation (red) [Kah09].

However, the visual control can detect the endosteum only after the exposure of the membrane. Therefore, laser pulses erroneously applied onto the critical structure are unavoidable in the following situation: suppose a single laser pulse can ablate $d\,\mu$m bone tissue while there exist some areas with only $d/2\,\mu$m overlying bone tissue. Unfortunately, without knowing that the bone layer is already critically thin, the control module will still classify these areas as "valid" and allow further pulses to be applied there. Consequently, after ablating the remaining $d/2\,\mu$m bone tissue, the rest energy of the laser pulse is completely applied onto the fragile endosteum, resulting in perforation on the structure (red area in the figure) accompanied by the high risk of perilymph leakage.

Residual Bone Thickness based Control: Conception Considering the critical situation above, it would be very advantageous if the position of the endosteum could be foresightedly detected before the exposure, based on which the thickness of the residual bone tissue can be measured. According to the obtained residual bone thickness profile, the controller can decide either to use a shorter pulse duration, resulting in less ablation depth, or even mark the position "invalid" if no shorter pulse is available, so that the ablation terminates locally for the involved region[2]. Thus, the safety of the fragile endosteum would be guaranteed.

Now, the question is: how to detect the position of the endosteum foresightedly before its exposure?

2.3.2 Foresighted Detection of Endosteum: How?

While developing laser-bone ablation systems, many researchers have confronted the similar situation like us, that is, how to automatically detect the boundary between the hard tissue and underlying soft tissue? During the last decade, several candidate sensor technologies for this purpose have been proposed.

One popular choice is to monitor the change of laser ablation induced emissions. As stated in section 2.2.2, the laser ablation is accompanied with audible micro-explosions. Due to the significantly different mechanical properties of hard and soft tissues, the acoustic emission induced by the micro-explosions on the two kinds of tissues is expected to be different. Therefore, some authors [LFG99, RSKW+04, SWK+07, LHLS07] have studied the feasibility of detecting the boundary by comparing the frequency spectra of the acoustic signal acquired during the ablation. The transition from hard tissue to underlying soft tissue is recognized by the change of the characteristic frequency bands.

Ruppert et al. [RTK+03, RTGW+04] have further investigated the possibility to detect the tissue boundary by measuring the intensity of the ablation plume (see figure 2.7a), where a drop of the intensity is the signal of tissue transition. However, a significant drawback of this kind of sensor technologies is that the boundary detection is only possible after the first pulse applied onto the soft tissue layer, which does not satisfy our requirement of a foresighted detection[3].

Alternatively, instead of detecting the position of the boundary directly, the current ablation depth can be online measured by ultra-

[2] For the later case, the residual bone layer is already thin enough and mechanically similar to soft tissue, which can be easily perforated manually by the surgeon. Detailed ablation strategy will be developed in section 5.4.

[3] The acoustic emission based approach will be discussed in detail in section 7.2.3.

sound [WSM+01, GTFP04] or confocal microscopy [SW10] etc. Thus, the residual bone thickness can be obtained by comparison between the current ablation depth with the total bone thickness measured from pre-operative CT or MRI. However, the accuracy of such an approach not only depends on the resolution of the measuring system itself, but also is limited by the accuracy of registration between the intra-operative measuring system and the pre-operative imaging as well as the relatively low resolution of CT and MRI that is more than 1/4 mm in general. Therefore, a direct bone thickness measurement is preferred. Another research [TPF09] reveals that such a measurement is possible using ultrasound. However, the technique provides currently an accuracy of only 0.4-0.6 mm, which is also not precise enough for our case. The fixation of ultrasound detector near the cochlea is also challenging.

Fortunately, there exists an emerging optical imaging technology, namely *optical coherence tomography* (OCT) [HSL+91, DF08], which provides a high resolution on micrometre scale and enables a contactless imaging of the internal micro-structures of biological tissue in-vivo. Hence, this sensor technology seems to match perfectly with the laser ablation. However, typical clinical application of this sensor technology is ophthalmology diagnosis or "optical biopsy" for soft tissues like arteries, nerves or skins. Would it be possible to use OCT to image the internal structure beneath the bony shell of cochlea and guide the ablation accordingly? Ohmi et al. [OTFH04] has stated the feasibility of using an OCT to observe the ablation process of biological tissues. Further researches [RBB03, UMA04, EWO+09, FSK+12, FKS+12] reveal that the OCT is able to show the internal structures beneath the surface of bone tissue. Therefore, the endosteum beneath the bone tissue would probably also be visible in OCT images, enabling the desired foresighted detection of the critical structure as well as the residual bone thickness based laser ablation control.

2.4 Conclusion

The conventional cochleostomy performed with burrs is a highly risky micro-surgery accompanied by trauma to the patient and a high demand on the skills and experiences of the surgeon. The precise laser ablation provides a perfect solution to these difficulties, where a precise closed-loop control of the ablation process to preserve the endosteum is however missing. With the resolution on micrometre scale, the contactless optical coherence tomography is a promising candidate for establishing the mandatory control loop, which is the main objective of this thesis and will be developed in the succeeding chapters.

CHAPTER 3

Optical Coherence Tomograhpy

Chosen as the sensor for online monitoring the laser-cochleostomy, the working principle of the optical coherence tomography will be introduced in this chapter. After a short description of the own OCT system, preliminary experiments are conducted to verify the feasibility of using OCT for the foresighted imaging of the critical cochlear endosteum. Finally, the control loop of the OCT guided laser-cochleostomy is proposed.

3.1 Working Principle of OCT

3.1.1 Introduction

Optical coherence tomography is an emerging non-invasive optical imaging modality in biomedical optics and medicine, which was invented by the workgroup of Fujumoto et al. [HSL$^+$91] in the early 1990's. OCT can provide real time cross-sectional imaging of the internal micro-structures in biological tissues. On most biological tissues, the imaging depth of OCT is up to a 2-3 mm while the resolution is typically 1-15 μm, which fills hence the gap between the confocal microscopy and ultrasonography, as illustrated in figure 3.1a.

OCT imaging, also known as *ultrasonography with light*, is analogous to ultrasonography except that it uses light instead of sound, which works with the pulse-echo mechanism: an incident measuring light beam (not necessarily a laser) is directed to the tissue sample and backscattered differently from structures that have varying optical properties, as well as from boundaries between structures. The deeper a structure is, the longer will the echo delay be (figure 3.1b).

By measuring these echoes and distributing their intensities according to their time delay, an *axial scan* (A-scan) that contains the information about the internal micro-structures along the measuring beam can be reconstructed, as illustrated in figure 3.1c. A global attenuating trend with the increasing depth can be observed from the A-scan due to the scattering and absorption of the light irradiation during the propagation.

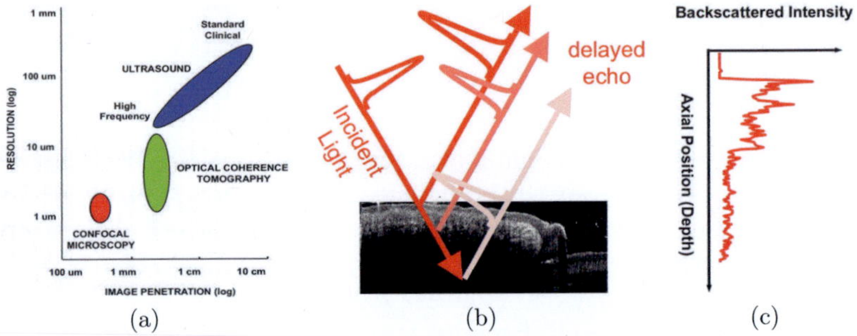

Figure 3.1: (a) Comparison of resolution and imaging depth for ultrasound, OCT and confocal microscopy [DF08]. (b) Basic working principle of OCT: ultrasonography with light, where the measuring beam directed to the target tissue is backscattered from different depths with different time delays and intensities (kindly provided by Wolfgang Wieser, chair for BioMolecular Optics at the University of Munich, Germany). (c) Illustration of intensity distribution along the incident beam in (b) [DF08].

Obviously, it is difficult to recognize structures from one-dimensional A-scans. In order to generate meaningful two-dimensional images, the measuring beam is translated along a transversal (X) direction (case 2D in figure 3.2), resulting in meaningful cross-sectional B-scans showing the internal micro-structures of the sample[1]. Further translation of the measuring beam in a raster pattern (XY) yields a three-dimensional volume accordingly (case 3D in figure 3.2). In the succeeding part of this thesis, the direction along the measuring beam (Z) and the other two scanning directions (XY) will be referred to as *axial direction* and *lateral direction* respectively.

[1] More example OCT images can be found in succeeding sections.

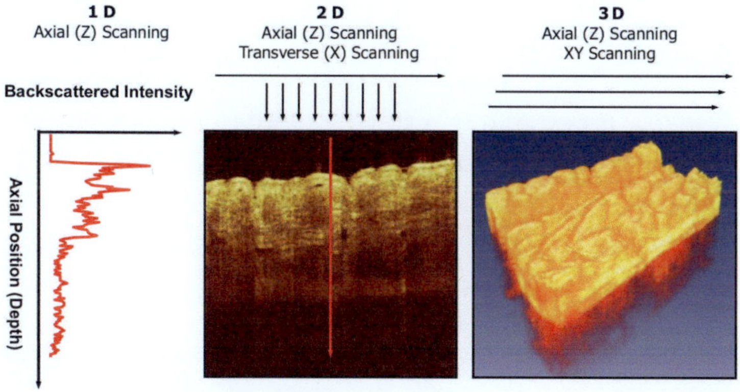

Figure 3.2: Generation of cross-sectional or three-dimensional images using OCT: cross-sectional images (2D) are generated by performing a series of axial scans at different transverse positions. Three-dimensional data sets (3D-OCT) can be generated by further raster scanning a series of two-dimensional data sets [DF08].

For a fast and precise translation of the measuring beam in the lateral directions, OCT systems are often equipped with the same kind of galvanometric scannershown in figure 2.8. Meanwhile, the scanner also enables a variable *scanning density*, which is defined as the number of A-scans per millimetre, resulting in an arbitrarily adjustable pixel size in lateral directions. Take advantage of this feature, any structure of interest could be dilated or compressed arbitrarily in the lateral direction for a more convenient observation, which is also useful for the critical structure detection developed later in section 5.3.

3.1.2 Time Domain OCT

Due to the extremely high velocity of light, the time delay of the echoes caused by a depth difference on micrometre scale is impossible to be resolved by the current technologies. Therefore, the OCT system does not really measure the time delay of the echoes. Instead, as its name suggests, the echo delay is measured by coherence of the incident and backscattered light. In the following, this principle is briefly explained with the simplest time domain OCT (TD-OCT), more details can be found in [Fuj01, Fuj06, DF08].

The main component of an OCT is a Michelson interferometer, in which the measuring beam from the light source is divided into two parts by a beam splitter. One of them is directed to the sample (*sample arm*) and the other part travels to a reference mirror (*reference arm*) whose position is adjustable, as illustrated in figure 3.3.

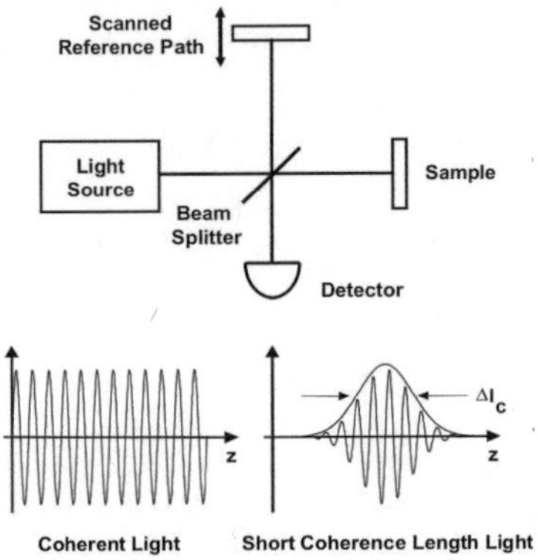

Figure 3.3: Illustration of time domain OCT [Fuj01].

An echo back reflected from some depth inside the sample travels back along the original path and then merges with the light coming back from the reference arm at the beam splitter. Supposing that the echo has travelled a distance of d_e and the reference light has travelled d_r. Both lights will be interfered if the difference between d_e and d_r is smaller than the **coherence length** of the light source, which is inversely proportional to the bandwidth of the light.

The time delay of the echo is then measured based on a classic optical measurement technique known as low-coherence interferometry, where a broad-bandwidth light source having a short coherence length is used. As a result, only the echoes satisfying $d_e \approx d_r$ can be interfered to the reference light. Meanwhile, as the path length d_r through the reference arm is already known, d_e can be hence intuitively obtained. The magnitudes and echo time delays of light along the whole A-scan can be then measured by scanning the reference arm and demodulating the interference signal intensity measured by the detector.

An important feature of OCT is, the axial resolution of the image is dominated by the coherence length of the light source. The broader the bandwidth of the light source is, the higher will the axial resolution be.

3.1.3 Fourier Domain OCT

In practice, the mechanical scanning part of the reference arm severely limits the speed of image acquisition. Fourier domain OCT (FD-OCT) [LHF$^+$03, DBCP$^+$03] was hence proposed, which has not only solved this problem, but also significantly improved the sensitivity of the system and provides much better image quality. The main difference of FD-OCT from TD-OCT is that the reference arm of FD-OCT is fixed, as illustrated in figure 3.4.

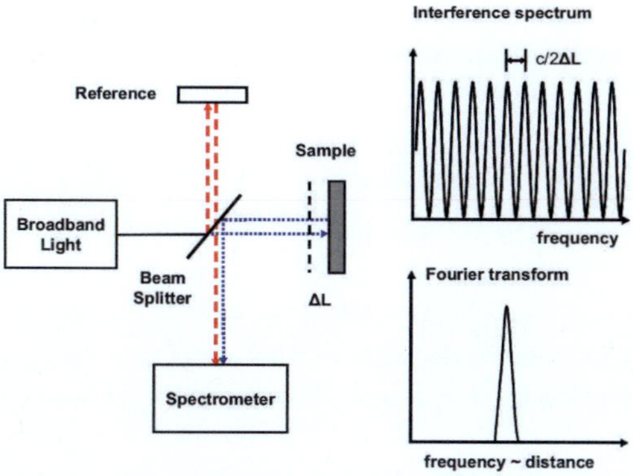

Figure 3.4: Illustration of Fourier domain OCT with fixed reference arm [DF08].

The imaging of FD-OCT is based on the fact that a Michelson interferometer acts like a periodic frequency filter, where the periodicity is a function of the path difference between the sample and reference arms. Taking the situation in figure 3.4 as example, suppose the path difference between the observed depth in the sample and the reference arms is $2\Delta L$. The constructive and destructive interferences will appear periodically every $c/2\Delta L$ with respect to the frequency of the measuring light (refer to [YY97, DiM12]), where c is the velocity of light. As a result, the interference spectrum is also periodic and its Fourier transform is an impulse at the corresponding depth[2]. A spectrometer is used as detector to measure the mixed interference spectra corresponding to all depths in the sample simultaneously. The Fourier transform of this interference spectra yields the A-scan in a single step.

[2] Be aware that the frequency in figure 3.4 denotes the frequency of the light, not the frequency of the periodic interference spectrum. The time domain and frequency domain of the Fourier transform in this case are "frequency of the measuring light" and "path length difference between sample and reference arms" respectively.

3.1.4 Swept Source-Fourier Domain OCT

As stated above, the light source of OCT must be broadband and low-coherent to enable the low-coherence interferometry, so that a narrow band light source such as laser is not capable for the OCT. In order to be able to use a narrow band light source, especially the laser which is much easier to be collimated and focused, the swept source-Fourier domain OCT (SS-OCT) was invented [CSYI03, YTdB+03].

A major characteristic of an SS-OCT is, although the light source is narrow band, its frequency is sweeping in time and covers a wide frequency band (figure 3.5). Actually, it can be regarded as a special case of FD-OCT. While FD-OCT generates the interference spectrum of all frequencies simultaneously (figure 3.4, top right), SS-OCT can measure only a single frequency each time.

By sweeping the frequency over the whole bandwidth in time (figure 3.5, top right), the interference spectrum with respect to time is generated (figure 3.5, bottom right). According to the frequency-time profile (figure 3.5, top right), the time axis of the spectrum in figure 3.5 bottom right can be mapped to frequency. Thus, the interference spectrum with respect to frequency same as FD-OCT (figure 3.4, top right) is obtained and the A-scan is calculated by Fourier transform as usual.

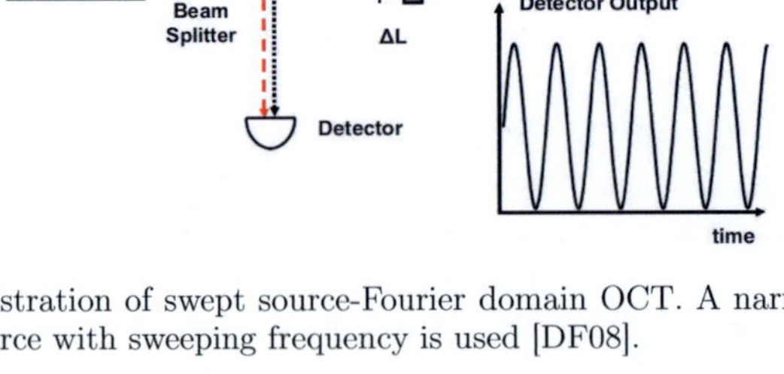

Figure 3.5: Illustration of swept source-Fourier domain OCT. A narrow band light source with sweeping frequency is used [DF08].

3.1.5 OCT System Setup

System Specifications Within the scope of this thesis, an in house built SS-OCT system is used to perform the OCT scans. A 54 kHz FDML-laser [HWF06, WPE+12] with a 104 nm tuning range (i.e. bandwidth) at a centre wavelength of 1310 nm is used as the light source. A Thorlabs GVS002 (Thorlabs GmbH, Dachau/Munich, Germany) galvanometric scanner (refer to figure 2.8) is installed to generate two- and three-dimensional OCT scans. The maximal scan angle of each mirror is ± 0.218 rad with an angular resolution of 15 μrad. The scanner is equipped with a focusing lens with a focal length of 75 mm, corresponding to the distance between the focal plane and the scanning system. The Rayleigh range of the measuring beam and axial resolution are 4.05 mm and 8.41 μm respectively.

Reconstruction of OCT A-Scan Giving the readings from the SS-OCT detector (figure 3.5), an OCT A-scan can be calculated by performing the following steps:

1. Background noise subtraction:
   Analogous to any other kind of electronic devices, OCT system also suffers from background noises induced by the hardware itself. Therefore, after system warming up or long time running, several scans are acquired without sample under the sample arm. The average background noise can be simply obtained by averaging them. For all the succeeding acquisition, the average background noise will be subtracted from the detector output.

2. Resampling:
   Due to the working mechanism, the sweeping velocity of the laser source is non-linear. The frequency-time profile is hence not a straight line shown in figure 3.5 top right but an S-shaped curve. Consequently, while mapping the equidistant time axis (figure 3.5 bottom right) to light frequency, the data points are no more equidistant and a Fourier transform is in this case impossible. Therefore, a linear interpolation is performed to the none equidistant data points in order to resample an equidistant data set.

3. Fourier transform:
   Performing the Fourier transform to the resampled data set, its magnitude of the resulting spectrum is exactly the A-scan.

4. Clipping:
   In order to increase the contrast of the image and make the pixel values additive instead of multiplicative, the A-scan is further logarithmized. According to the user specified upper and lower boundaries of the dynamic range, all values larger than the upper boundary are set to 255, while those smaller than the lower boundary are set to 0. The other values are linearly distributed between 0-255. A gray scale A-scan is thereby reconstructed.

3.2 Feasibility Study

Before starting the development of the closed-loop control of the laser-cochleostomy, preliminary experiments were conducted to examine the feasibility of using OCT for monitoring the bottom of the cochleostomy. The following two points will play a decisive role, whether OCT is capable of predicting the position of the cochlear endosteum or not:

- Is cochlear endosteum indeed visible in OCT images?
- What is the OCT imaging depth in cochlea?

3.2.1 Cochlear Endosteum in OCT Image

Formalin Fixed Human Cochlea To answer the first question, a formalin fixed human cochlea was isolated from a cadaver (figure 3.6a), on which an insertion channel was drilled with a diamond burr to simulate the process of the cochleostomy[3]. OCT scans were acquired at different phases during the drilling process with different channel depths.

Due to the attenuating intensity of the echo with the increasing depth (see section 3.1.1), the cochlear endosteum is not visible in the OCT scans acquired at the early stage of the drilling process while the overlaying bone tissue still has the thickness of more than one millimetre. Nevertheless, with the increasing channel depth, the bone layer gets thinner and thinner. More and more measuring light can reach the critical structure. In the OCT scans acquired during the end phase of the drilling process, the membrane can be clearly seen (figure 3.6b).

[3] The author wants to thank the project partners from Department of Oto-Rhino-Laryngology, University Hospital Düsseldorf, Germany for providing the specimens.

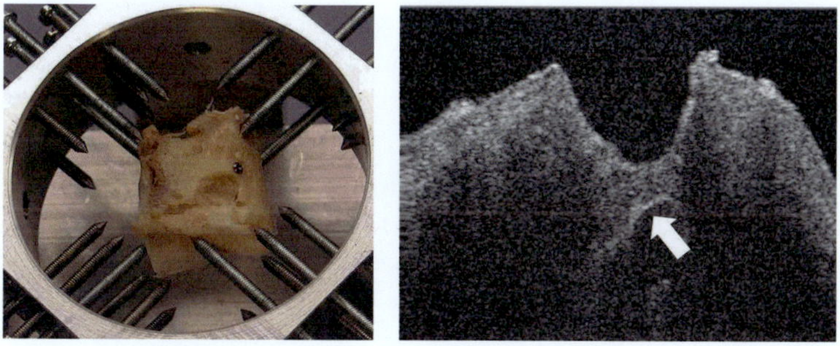

(a) (b)

Figure 3.6: (a) A formalin fixed human cochlea isolated from a cadaver and (b) an OCT scan acquired during the end phase of cochleostomy on it. The cochlear endosteum can be clearly observed (arrow).

Fresh Porcine Cochlea With the concern that formalin might have changed the optical properties of the observed tissue, which might make the originally invisible structures to be visible, further experiments were conducted with freshly isolated porcine cochlea (figure 3.7a). The bone thickness near the apex (the centre of the snail-shaped spiral of cochlea) is less than 100 μm and nearly half transparent, so that the snail-shaped structure can even be observed directly without OCT.

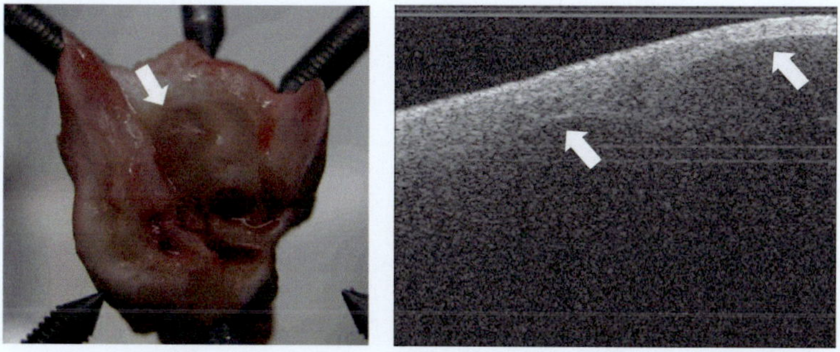

(a) (b)

Figure 3.7: (a) A freshly isolated porcine cochlea. OCT scans are acquired near its apex (arrow) without drilling. (b) An OCT scan of the apex, where two scalae can be observed and endosteum is also visible (arrows).

OCT scans were acquired on the original surface of the cochlea near the apex without drilling. The endosteum beneath the bone tissue can be clearly seen near the apex (arrow on the right in figure 3.7b), which gets less visible (arrow on the left figure 3.7b) and finally disappears towards the base of the cochlea with the increasing bone thickness. This contradicts the above concern of altered optical properties due to formalin.

Influence of Tissue Layer with Thermal Injury As introduced in section 2.2.2, a thin tissue layer with thermal injury may be formed on the bottom of the laser ablated channel. In order to investigate whether this layer may have any negative influences on the OCT imaging, divers craters with different radii and depths were ablated with the CO_2 laser on the porcine cochlea and OCT scans of these craters were acquired, as shown in figure 3.8.

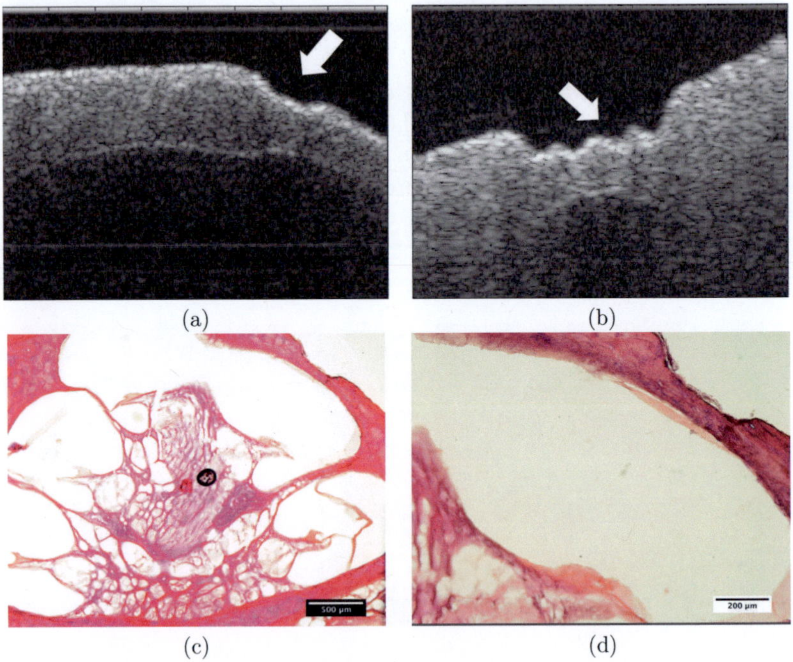

Figure 3.8: (a-b) OCT scans of laser ablated craters (arrows) with different size and depths on fresh porcine cochleae. The cochlear endosteum is visible beneath the craters. (c-d) The corresponding histology of scan (a) under (c) 4x and (d) 10x magnification (gratefully provided by Mr.Marcel Weller from Department of Oto-Rhino-Laryngology, University Hospital Düsseldorf, Germany), where a very thin layer of carbonised tissue can be observed on the bottom of the crater.

It can be observed that the endosteum is still visible beneath the craters, which indicates that the injured tissue layer has no significant negative influences on the OCT imaging of the cochlear endosteum.[4]

3.2.2 OCT Imaging Depth in Compact Bone

From the experiments in section 3.2.1 we conclude that the OCT is capable of detecting the cochlear endosteum, however, with a precondition: the overlying bone tissue has to be thin enough. This leads to the second question at the beginning of the section 3.2. In other words, how many micrometres in advance can OCT detect the critical structure? In our case, an earlier detection of the critical structure is desired.

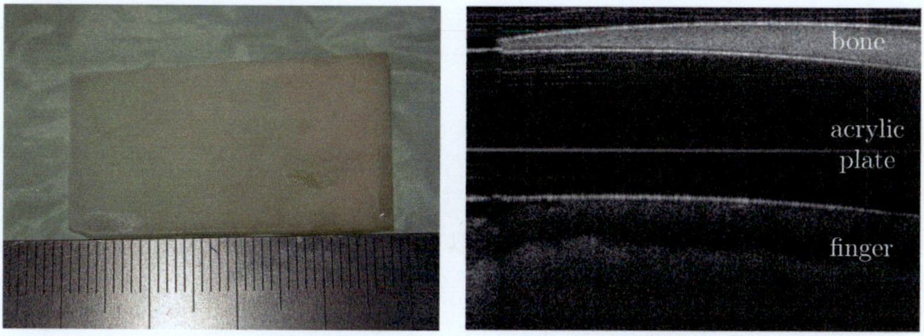

(a) (b)

Figure 3.9: (a) A manually polished wedge-shaped bovine bone sheet whose thickness increases from 0.1 mm at the left edge to 1.6 mm at the right edge and (b) the OCT scan of its left part acquired with an acrylic plate and finger underneath.

In order to estimate the maximal OCT imaging depth in cochlea, a native bovine compact bone sheet (separated from femur, shown in figure 3.9a) was manually polished to be wedge-shaped, which consists of the same kind of bone material as cochlea. The thickness of the sheet varies from 0.1 mm at its left edge to 1.6 mm at the right edge linearly over a range of circa 38 mm. Through very simple geometric calculation the thickness at any given point on the specimen can be obtained with the accuracy of several tens micrometres.

[4] It can be observed that the shape of the endosteum looks discontinuous under the craters in figure 3.8a, while this structure is actually a smooth one (figure 3.8c-d). This is not caused by the tissue layer with thermal injury but an inherent artefact of OCT due to different speed of light in bone and air. This artefact will be handled in more detail in section 5.1.3.4.

The bone specimen was fixed on a transparent acrylic plate and OCT scans were acquired with finger underneath (figure 3.9b). It can be clearly observed that on the left side of the image where the bone is thinner, the bone-acrylic and acrylic-finger boundaries are sharper than on the right side[5]. By scanning towards the right side, the OCT imaging depth into compact bone tissue is determined to be 500-800 μm.

3.3 Conclusion

Being able to image the cochlear endosteum about half a millimetre in advance, meanwhile providing a high resolution on micrometre scale, OCT is very capable of monitoring the laser-cochleostomy. By analysing the OCT images properly, the position of the critical structure could be determined. Thus, the residual bone thickness based control concept conceived in section 2.3.1 becomes possible and the following control loop is designed accordingly.

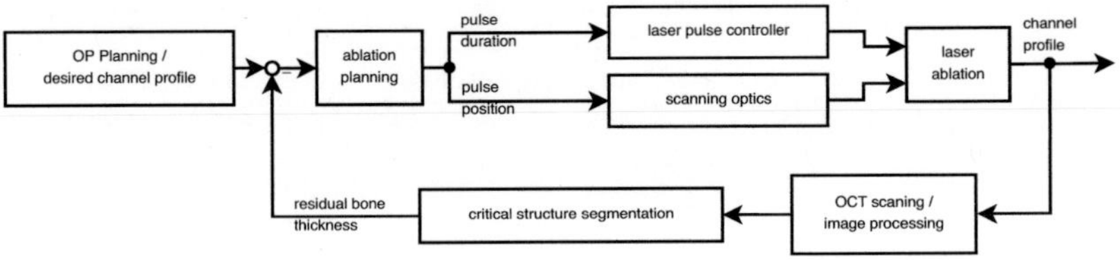

Figure 3.10: Design of the control loop of the OCT guided laser-cochleostomy.

During the process of OCT guided laser-cochleostomy, the laser ablation and OCT scanning are performed alternately. After each round of ablation, a three-dimensional OCT volume scan of the cochleostomy is acquired. If the position of the bone-endosteum- perilymph boundary could be detected after proper image processing, the residual bone thickness above this critical structure can be calculated. Based on the obtained bone thickness distribution, the pulse positions and pulse durations for the next round of laser ablation are planned by a computer algorithm. The ablation parameters are then transmitted to the corresponding control modules and the ablation pattern is executed. By repeating this procedure until the critical structure is reached, the desired endosteum preserving cochleostomy can be achieved.

[5] It can also be noticed that the surface of the bone specimen and acrylic plate are curved in the OCT image, which is another artefact of OCT. It will be handled in more detail in section 5.1.2.

CHAPTER 4

Image Segmentation

Obviously, image segmentation will play a very important role in the endosteum detection in OCT images. Before proceeding to develop the control loop proposed in figure 3.10, a short excursion will be made in this chapter to review the background knowledges in this field that are necessary for the succeeding development.

4.1 Spatial Domain Operations

Generally, image segmentation requires a pre-processing to enhance the image, so that features can be emphasised and noises are suppressed. Image enhancement approaches can be classified into two categories: spatial domain and frequency domain methods. The spatial domain methods focus on manipulating the image pixels directly while the frequency domain methods are based on processing the Fourier transform of the whole image. In this thesis, only the spatial domain methods are used. An operation in the spatial domain can be formally described as

$$g(x, y) = T[f(x, y)] \tag{4.1}$$

where f is the input image and g is the processed image; T is an operator on f defined over some neighbourhood of the pixel (x, y). In most cases, the neighbourhood is defined to be rectangular with odd size due to the ease of implementation. The simplest form of T is the pixel-wise operation (also known as gray scale transformation), i.e. the neighbourhood has a size of 1×1. An example is the clipping operation while reconstructing the A-scan (section 3.1.5).

Operations defined over larger neighbourhood often provide more flexibility, which can be used for smoothing, sharpening the image as well as feature extraction etc. The most important operation of this kind is the so called *linear spatial filtering*. The filtering of an $M \times N$ image f using an $m \times n$ filter mask w is defined by the following equation, where $a = (m-1)/2$ and $b = (n-1)/2$:

$$g(x,y) = \sum_{s=-a}^{a} \sum_{t=-b}^{b} w(s,t) f(x+s, y+t) \tag{4.2}$$

which is actually the discrete form of cross-correlation between the image and the mask. By defining proper filter mask w, diverse enhancements can be realised, which are often the first step of diverse segmentation techniques. Some important filters are stated in the following.

Smoothing Filter Smoothing filters are used for blurring the image and for noise reduction. The most common ones are the averaging filter and Gaussian filter:

$$\frac{1}{9} \cdot \begin{pmatrix} 1 & 1 & 1 \\ 1 & 1 & 1 \\ 1 & 1 & 1 \end{pmatrix} \qquad \frac{1}{16} \cdot \begin{pmatrix} 1 & 2 & 1 \\ 2 & 4 & 2 \\ 1 & 2 & 1 \end{pmatrix} \tag{4.3}$$

where the left one is a 3×3 average filter and the right one is the discrete form of a Gaussian function in a 3×3 neighbourhood.

Sharpening Filter Sharpening filters can highlight fine image details and are often used for emphasising the boundaries between objects in the image. Basic idea of these filters is to calculate the derivatives of the image in a discrete form, for example the Sobel operators:

$$\begin{pmatrix} -1 & -2 & -1 \\ 0 & 0 & 0 \\ 1 & 2 & 1 \end{pmatrix} \qquad \begin{pmatrix} -1 & 0 & 1 \\ -2 & 0 & 2 \\ -1 & 0 & 1 \end{pmatrix}. \tag{4.4}$$

where the left one is the vertical and right one is the horizontal first order derivatives respectively, denote as G_{vert} and G_{hori} in the following, which are often used for extracting horizontal and vertical boundaries in the image. In practice, the magnitude of the gradient $\nabla f = (G_{\text{hori}}, G_{\text{vert}})$ is also used quite often, which is approximated by

$$|\nabla f| \approx |G_{\text{vert}}| + |G_{\text{hori}}| \tag{4.5}$$

so that an inefficient calculation of the square root $|\nabla f| = (G_{\text{hori}}^2 + G_{\text{vert}}^2)^{1/2}$ can be avoided. Meanwhile, the second order derivatives are calculated with the Laplacian operator, which are defined as

$$\begin{pmatrix} 0 & 1 & 0 \\ 1 & -4 & 1 \\ 0 & 1 & 0 \end{pmatrix} \qquad \begin{pmatrix} 1 & 0 & 1 \\ 0 & -4 & 0 \\ 1 & 0 & 1 \end{pmatrix} \qquad \begin{pmatrix} 1 & 1 & 1 \\ 1 & -8 & 1 \\ 1 & 1 & 1 \end{pmatrix} \tag{4.6}$$

where the left one is used to extract horizontal and vertical boundaries while the middle one is capable of detecting the diagonal edges. The one on the right is the sum of the other two filters and can detect boundaries in all four directions simultaneously. Considering that the second order derivatives are sensible to noises, Gaussian filter is often applied before the Laplacian to smooth the image, known as the Laplacian of Gaussian.

Median Filter Unlike the linear spacial filters, median filter belongs to a filter category called *order-statistics filters* which are non-linear. Such filters are based on ordering the pixels inside the neighbourhood encompassed by the filter and replacing the value of the centre pixel with the value determined by the ordering result.

The median filter, as its name implies, replaces the centre pixel with the median of all pixels within the neighbourhood. It is particularly effective for suppressing impulse noises and meanwhile brings considerably less blurring effect than the linear smoothing filters introduced above [GW02]. After applying an appropriate filter chain consists of divers filters, the image with suppressed noises and enhanced boundaries are ready to be segmented.

4.2 Image Segmentation: State of the Art

Segmentation is one of the most important topic in image processing, which is the partitioning of an image or volume into constituent regions that are meaningful for a specific task. For example, the region between the most superficial air-bone boundary and the cochlear endosteum in figures 3.6-3.8 are exactly the bone layer that should be ablated.

Although the topic has been intensively studied for decades, image segmentation remains a difficult task due to tremendous variability of object shapes and the variation in image quality. There exists hence no universal image segmentation techniques. Generally, the main image segmentation techniques can be divided into three categories: basic segmentation, deformable models based segmentation and segmentation by morphological watersheds, where the basic segmentation can be again subdivided into thresholding, region-based and edge-based segmentation. In the following, a brief overview of these techniques will be given, details can be found in [GW02, FS00].

4.2.1 Basic Segmentation

Thresholding Thresholding is a simple but effective segmentation method. By defining a gray value threshold, a given image I can be divided into two parts with pixels brighter than the threshold as foreground and darker ones as background, or even more parts by multiple thresholds. The thresholds are typically estimated from the histogram of gray values of pixels in the image, for example the Otsu algorithm [Ots79] that maximizes the inter-class variance and minimizes the intra-class variance of the two pixel classes separated by the threshold. Moreover, the threshold must not be uniform for the whole image but can be spatially adaptive to the local image properties, for example the Chow and Kaneko thresholding [CK72].

Region-Based Segmentation Region-based approaches, including region growing and region split-and-merge algorithms, distinguish regions in the given image based on some homogeneity properties directly. Uniformity criteria are predefined in order to determine whether the chosen pixels have similar properties (such as gray value, colour, texture etc.) or not. As its name implies, the region growing algorithm starts with a set of seed points. For each region to be segmented, pixels neighbouring to the seeds are appended to the seeds set if they meet the uniformity criteria, until no more neighbouring pixels with similar properties can be found.

Split-and-merge algorithm has two steps: region split and region merge. Region split works exactly the opposite to the region growing. If the pixels within a region does not satisfy the uniformity criteria, the region will be divided into 4 sub-images (8 for three-dimensional volume) recursively until the uniformity criteria are met in each sub-region. The region merge is similar as region growing, where the sub-regions of the same parent region and adjacent sub-regions of different parents satisfying the uniformity criteria are unified.

Edge-Based Segmentation Edge-based approaches segment the images by detecting the boundaries between different regions. The set of candidate boundary pixels $\{b_i\}$ is extracted by applying the spatial filtering introduced in section 4.1 and comparing the resulting edge magnitude $|e(b_i)|$ denoting the possibility that b_i is an boundary pixel with some thresholds. These candidates are linked appropriately afterwards in order to generate boundaries.

In practice, if the boundary to be detected is a parametric curve or surface (e.g. straight line, circle, ellipse, sphere, ellipsoid etc.), (generalized) *Hough Transform* [Hou62, Bal81] is a powerful tool for the linking. However, the structures in medical images are often not parametric ones, like the most superficial air-bone interface in the OCT images shown in figure 3.6b and figure 3.8. The basic solution for linking the edge pixels in such cases is the so called *border tracing* algorithm, where two successive candidate boundary pixels b_j and b_{j+1} will be connected if the following feasibility constraints hold:

$$\begin{cases} |e(b_j) - e(b_{j+1})| < T_1 & \text{(4.7a)} \\ |\phi(b_j) - \phi(b_{j+1})| \bmod 2\pi < T_2 & \text{(4.7b)} \end{cases}$$

where T_1, T_2 are predetermined thresholds and $\phi(b_i)$ is the edge orientation at b_i produced by the applied filters. The inequality (4.7a) guarantees that the edge magnitude along the resulting boundary will be relatively uniform and (4.7b) prevents a sudden change of the edge orientation, resulting in a smooth curve. Generally, for a given candidate pixel b_i, there exist often more than one neighbours b_{i+1} satisfying these inequalities.

In order to obtain a curve that is globally optimal in some sense over its entire length, graph based algorithms are the common choices. The segmentation problem can be converted to graph problems such as minimum-cost path, minimum-cost closed set, minimum cut [GW14] etc. The simplest way to construct a graph is to regard the pixels b_i as vertices and the 2-tuples $E(b_i, b_j)$ as the edges of the graph if b_i and b_j are neighbouring pixels. The edge magnitude such as gray value gradient from b_i to b_j is assigned to $E(b_i, b_j)$ as its weight. A maximum cut of the graph is then exactly the boundary to be detected. However, this approach is only suitable for the relatively simple situation in which the search for the boundaries can be done in one dimension.

For more complicated situations, the design of the graph is more challenging. An example is the detection of edge-weak surfaces in three-dimensional OCT volumes such as the retinal layers in human eyes (figure 4.1), which can be solved by a novel graph based approach Curvature-UnBounded Optimal Smooth Surface (CuBOSS) [XSD+11, XSZ+11, XSD+12] proposed by the work group of Zonka et al.

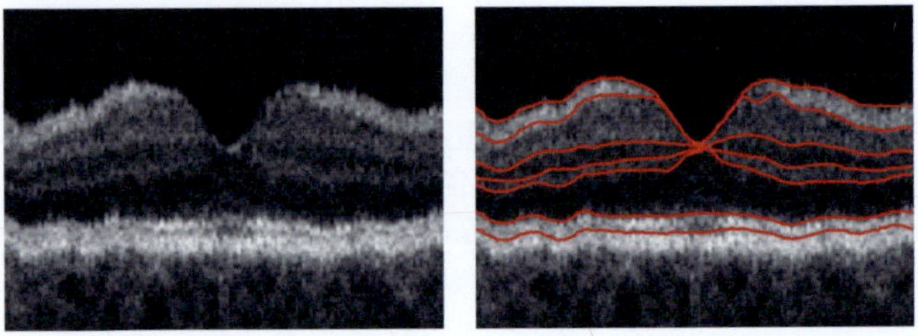

(a) (b)

Figure 4.1: Segmentation of multiple retinal layer boundaries in OCT images using CuBOSS algorithm: (a) the original image and (b) the detected boundaries [HWA+07].

CuBOSS constructs the graph as following: for a single frame in the OCT volume, each vertex is a 3-tuple $V(u, c, b)$, where u, c and b are pixels in successive A-scans. u, c and b satisfy that the vertical distance between (u, c) and (c, b) are smaller than N pixels, where N is a user defined threshold. This constrain is similar to equation (4.7b) in order to limit the curvature of the resulting boundary. The cost of the vertex is defined as following:

$$\text{cost}(V(u, c, b)) = \alpha\,|\kappa(V(u, c, b))| + (1 - \alpha)w(c) \tag{4.8}$$

where $\kappa(V(u, c, b))$ is the discrete curvature of the curve at c determined by the position of (u, c, b); $w(c)$ represents the inverse of the probability that c is a boundary pixel, for example the inverse of the absolute gray value gradient $1/|\nabla I(c)|$. The boundary to be detected in each frame is corresponding to the minimum-cost path in the graph and can be determined using dynamic programming or Dijkstra's algorithm [Dij59].

The ratio $0 \leq \alpha \leq 1$ in equation (4.8) is manually determined and a larger α will result in a smoother curve with lower curvature. The detected boundaries in single frames are connected as a surface. A second graph is constructed similarly in the perpendicular direction of the frame to obtain an optimal surface in the sense of low mean curvature.

Although the graph based approach permits the determination of globally optimal boundaries, the computational cost is very high. The order of the graph (number of vertices) is at least the same as the size of the volume. For special case like CuBOSS, N^2 vertices are added to the graph for each single voxel. Therefore, extra optimization for the efficiency is required while implementing the graph-based approaches.

4.2.2 Deformable Models Based Segmentation

In particular, medical images are often corrupted by noises and artefacts. Many important structures are therefore edge-weak in the images. In OCT images, the structures beneath the tissue surface are often not clear enough with the increasing depth, for example the internal retina layers in figure 4.1 and the cochlear endosteum with relatively thick overlying bone layer in figure 3.7b.

As a result, the simple theresholding, region growing, edge detection may often fail to detect the relevant boundaries correctly. The edge linking using Hough transform works only for parametric boundaries while the graph based approaches are inefficient. To overcome these difficulties, *deformable models* have been extensively studied, which can provide promising results with relatively high efficiency and is widely applied in medical image segmentation.

Parametric Deformable Models The concept of deformable models was first introduced by Terzopoulos [Ter80, TF88]. On initialization, an estimation of the boundary position is given, which will be deformed in the succeeding steps to minimize the sum of internal and external energy along the extracted curve (surface in three-dimensional case).

The internal energies are properties of the detected curve itself and are designed to keep the curve smooth during deformation; the external energies are computed from image data or even added by the user to deform the curve toward the object boundaries or other desired features in the image. The minimization of the energy is generally solved by numerical approximation of the corresponding Euler-Lagrange differential equations using finite difference method (FDM) or finite element method (FEM).

The most famous and successful deformable model is the active contour model *snake* [KWT88], where the internal and external energies along the detected curve c are defined by the following equation:

$$E_{\text{snake}} = \frac{1}{2}\int_c (E_{\text{int}} + E_{\text{ext}})\mathrm{d}s \tag{4.9}$$

with $E_{\text{int}} = \alpha(s)\left|\frac{\partial c(s)}{\partial s}\right|^2 + \beta(s)\left|\frac{\partial^2 c(s)}{\partial s^2}\right|^2$ and $E_{\text{ext}} = -\gamma(s)|\nabla I(s)|^2$

where the first and second order derivatives of c are the tangent vector and principle normal vector of the detected curve at the position s respectively. Their magnitude denote the local tension and bending energy [BP94]. The external energy E_{ext} is the gradient of the gray value at $c(s)$ and the negative weight $-\gamma(s)$ indicates that pixels with high gray value gradient are more likely to be located on the boundary.

However, the external energy given by equation (4.9) often converges to local minimums and is not able to deform the contour into boundary concavities if the initialization is far from the actual position of the boundary. Xu et al. hence replaced the simple gradient term with a vector diffusion equation that diffuses the gradient into regions distant from the boundary [XP97], yielding a *gradient vector flow* (GVF) field, as illustrated in figure 4.2a.

For concrete applications, extra artificial energy terms are often designed specifically according to the situation and added to the external energy to further constrain the deformation of the contour. For example, Fuchs et al. [FSK$^+$12] defined an vertical pressure term $\vec{n} = (0, \pm 1\text{px})$ to deform the boundary in the vertical direction along the A-scans (figure 4.2b). After applying the adapted snake model to each single frame in the OCT volume, Fuchs et al. reconstructed the 3D profile of the bone surface by combining the obtained curves together according to the coordinates of the frames. Alternatively, the two-dimensional active contour model can also be extended to three-dimensional cases to approximate the complete 3D surface profile directly, known as *deformable surface model* [CCA92, MT99, DYQS04].

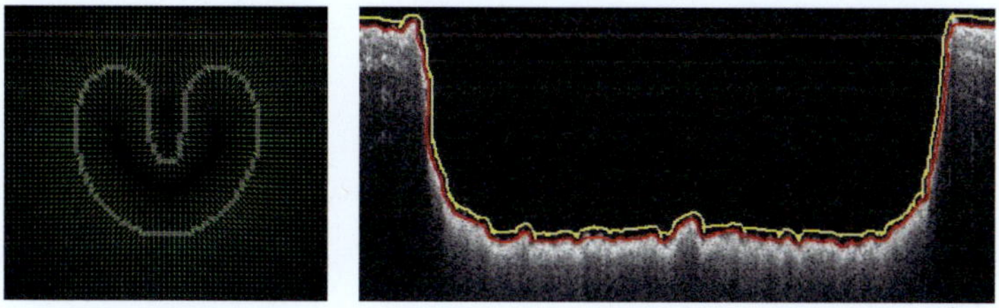

(a) (b)

Figure 4.2: (a) An example of gradient vector flow field [XP97], where all vectors are pointing to the U-shaped contour. (b) Segmentation of bone surface in OCT scan using snake model, where the yellow curve is the initialization and the red one is the final result after deformation [FSK$^+$12].

Providing a more stable result comparing with the basic segmentation, the main disadvantage of parametric deformable models is that no deterministic method exists for choosing the optimal weights of the energy terms in the cost function such as the α, β and γ in equation (4.9). These parameters are determined either empirically by user or using training sets if the to be segmented structure has some special properties. Moreover, an appropriate initialization of the model is also necessary to achieve a good segmentation result.

Active Shape Models *Active shape model* (ASM) is another important deformable model proposed by Cootes et al. [CT92, CTCG95, CET98], which works in a quite different way from the parametric deformable models by means of incorporating A-prior shape information of the structure to be detected.

The A-prior model of ASM is constructed by the so called *Point Distribution Model*, where a training set with n images is given. In addition, m feature points or landmarks on the structure to be detected are labelled in each training image, for example the 114 landmarks in the MR brain image shown in figure 4.3a. Denoting the coordinates of the m landmarks in the i-th training data by[1] $\mathbf{x}_i = (x_1, y_1, \ldots, x_m, y_m)^T$, the

[1] $\mathbf{x}_i = (x_1, y_1, z_1, \ldots, x_m, y_m, z_m)^T$ for three-dimensional volumes.

mean shape of the structure is defined as the arithmetic average of the n images $\bar{\mathbf{x}} = \sum_{i=1}^{n} \mathbf{x}_i / n$. The covariance matrix S of the training set is computed by

$$S = \frac{1}{n-1} \sum_{i=1}^{n} (\mathbf{x}_i - \bar{\mathbf{x}}) \cdot (\mathbf{x}_i - \bar{\mathbf{x}})^T$$

Calculating the eigenvectors $\{\phi_1, \ldots, \phi_t\}$ corresponding to the most significant t eigenvalues, which characterize almost the entire variability of the training set. In general, t is much smaller than the number of points m in the point distribution model. Consequently, any shape $\mathbf{x}$ in the training set can be approximated by the *principal component analysis*

$$\mathbf{x} \approx \bar{\mathbf{x}} + \Phi \cdot \mathbf{b} \tag{4.10}$$

where $\Phi = (\phi_1 | \phi_2 | \ldots | \phi_t)$ is the matrix composed of the t eigenvectors and $\mathbf{b} = (b_1, b_2, \ldots, b_t)^T$ is the weight vector of the eigenvectors, referred to as the *shape parameters.* The model can be deformed by changing the weights in $\mathbf{b}$ within some reasonable limits to constrain the deformation.

The segmentation of the desired structure is determined iteratively by initializing the active shape model $\mathbf{x} = \bar{\mathbf{x}}$. In each succeeding iteration, a global least squares fitting is first performed to adjust the position, orientation and scaling of the model $\mathbf{x}$ to align it to the given image. The deformation of the model $\mathrm{d}\mathbf{x}$ is then obtained by comparing the current status of $\mathbf{x}$ with the result of the least squares fitting. The change of the shape parameters $\mathrm{d}\mathbf{b}$ is computed by

$$\mathrm{d}\mathbf{b} = \Phi^{-1} \mathrm{d}\mathbf{x} = \Phi^T \mathrm{d}\mathbf{x}$$

Substituting new shape parameters $\mathbf{b}' = \mathbf{b} + \mathrm{d}\mathbf{b}$ into equation (4.10), the new active shape model $\mathbf{x}'$ for the next iterationis obtained. Repeating the above iterations until the difference between $\mathbf{x}'$ and $\mathbf{x}$ is insignificant. Figure 4.3b-d show an example of applying the ASM to detect the atrium in echocardiogram.

The main advantage of using such an A-priori knowledge based approach is that even the structure to be detected is only partially visible, for instance the upper part of the atrium in figure 4.3b has no clear boundary, the algorithm is still able to give an estimation of the boundary position. However, a large training set is necessary for establishing the point distribution model of the ASM for every particular application. The automatic labelling of the feature points $\{\mathbf{x}_i\}$ in the training set is often challenging as well.

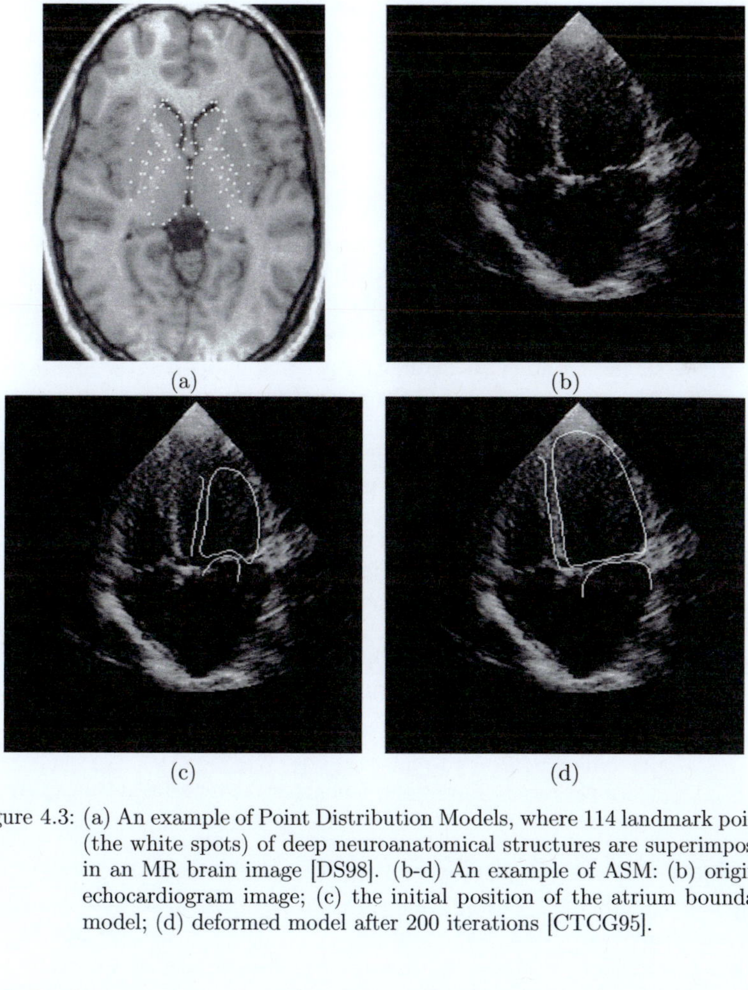

Figure 4.3: (a) An example of Point Distribution Models, where 114 landmark points (the white spots) of deep neuroanatomical structures are superimposed in an MR brain image [DS98]. (b-d) An example of ASM: (b) original echocardiogram image; (c) the initial position of the atrium boundary model; (d) deformed model after 200 iterations [CTCG95].

4.2.3 Segmentation by Morphological Watersheds

Morphological watersheds provides a stable segmentation in a quite different way from the above introduced methods. The basic concept is to regard the input image as a topographic map where the gray values or gradients of the pixels represent the sea level elevation of points (figure 4.4a and b). The points in the topographic map can be divided into three classes: (i) regional minimum; (ii) point, where a drop of water falls on it will fall with certainty to a single regional minimum; (iii) point, where a drop of water falls on it will fall into multiple regional minimums with equal probabilities. The points of class iii form the *watershed lines.*

The segmentation works by means of flooding the topographic map by letting water level in all regions rise uniformly. When the water in distinct regions is about to merge, an infinite high dam is built between the regions to avoid the merging (figure 4.4c), which is corresponding to the watershed line. Rising the water level continuously until only the dams are visible above the water line, the algorithm terminates and the resulting watershed lines are exactly the boundaries partitioning the image. Markers associated with objects of interest and background are often set to the regions to avoid the phenomenon *over-segmentation*, where the image is partitioned into too many regions.

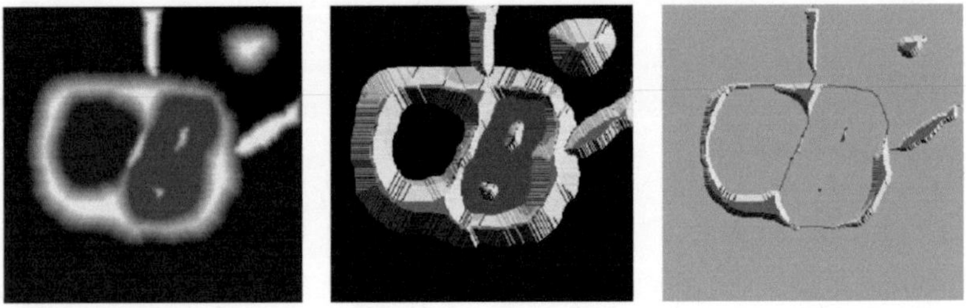

(a) (b) (c)

Figure 4.4: (a-b) Concept of morphological watersheds: (a) the input image and (b) the corresponding topographic map. (c) Dams are built to avoid merging of distinct regions during the flooding of the topographic map [GW02].

Implementation In practice, the process of flooding the topographic map is implemented by morphological operations, which are based on the set theory. Besides, two additional definitions which do not belong to basic set theory are needed, namely the *translation* of a set B:

$$(B)_z = \{c | c = b + z, \forall b \in B\}$$

and its *reflection*

$$\hat{B} = \{w | w = -b, \forall b \in B\}$$

There are two primitive morphological operations, *dilation* and *erosion*, which are defined as

$$\begin{cases} A \oplus B = \{z | (\hat{B})_z \cap A \neq \emptyset\} \\ A \ominus B = \{z | (B)_z \subseteq A\} \end{cases}$$

Commonly, the set B is often referred to as the *structuring element* in these operations, whose shape can be chosen according to the particular applications individually. Figure 4.5 illustrates the expanding effect of dilation and shrinking effect of erosion operations applied to a shape A with a disk structuring element B.

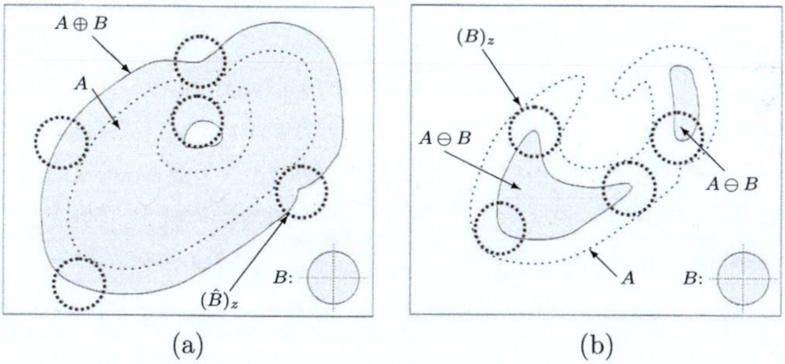

Figure 4.5: The effect of (a) dilation and (b) erosion of shape A with structuring element B [FS00].

The flooding procedure of the morphological watersheds can be then regarded as a dilation operation with a 3×3 symmetric rectangular structuring element. In other words, the regions are expanded for the width of one pixel in each flooding step. After the dilation, the overlapping pixels of two distinct regions are located on watershed lines separating the two regions.

4.3 Morphological Surface Smoothing

The morphological operations can be applied not only for the segmentation itself, but also for the post-processing of the segmented regions, for example skeleton extraction, boundary extraction, region filling, convex hull determination etc (details refer to [FS00, GW02]). For our case, the smoothing effect of morphological operations is useful for post-processing (see figure 5.12 and relevant texts).

Two further morphological operations are essential for this purpose, namely the *opening* operation

$$A \circ B = (A \ominus B) \oplus B \tag{4.11}$$

and the *closing* operation

$$A \bullet B = (A \oplus B) \ominus B \tag{4.12}$$

The effect of applying morphological opening and closing operations to shape A with a disk structuring element B is illustrated in figure 4.6a-b, where the two tips of shape A are eliminated after the opening operation and the gap between them are filled after the closing operation. This phenomenon indicates that the morphological opening and closing can be used to remove sharp peaks and to fill narrow gaps in a region if the structuring element is chosen properly.

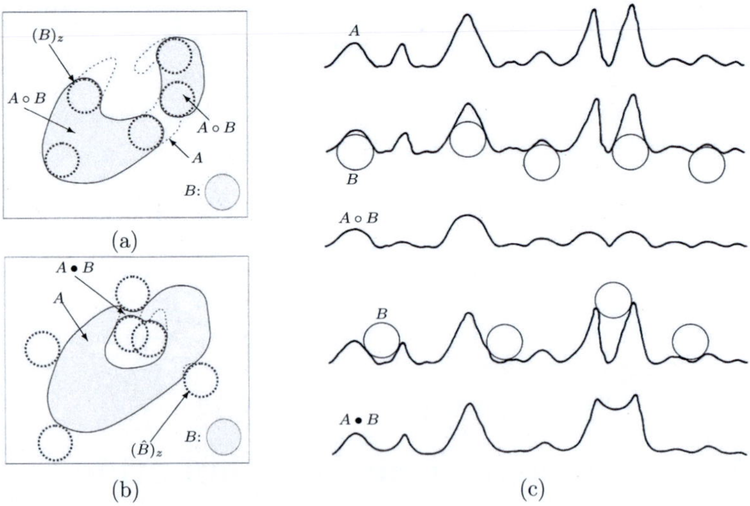

Figure 4.6: (a-b) The effect of (a) opening and (b) closing of shape A with structuring element B [FS00]. (c) Principle of gray-scale opening and closing of gray-scale line A with structuring element B, which are corresponding to rolling the structuring element B over A from the upper and lower sides respectively [GW02].

Particularly, an $M \times N$ three-dimensional surface of an object can be regarded as an $M \times N$ gray scale image. The surface smoothing problem can be then solved by applying the gray scale opening and closing illustrated in figure 4.6c, which can be understood as rolling the structuring element over the lower (for opening) and upper (for closing) sides of the surface. By choosing a proper radius of the structuring element, a smooth surface profile without sharp peaks and gaps can be obtained.

CHAPTER 5

Detection of Cochlear Endosteum

The feasibility study in section 3.2 indicates that OCT is a promising candidate of monitoring the channel bottom during the process of laser-cochleostomy. The key issue of establishing the desired closed-loop control of the laser ablation is now:

How to detect the position of the cochlear endosteum in three dimensional OCT volumes and how to guide the ablating laser accordingly?

In this chapter, a solution to this question will be provided. As the first step, artefacts in OCT images that may hinder the detection of the tissue boundary are studied and corresponding algorithms for artefact correction are developed accordingly. Then we focus on enhancing the image quality of the OCT scans and a novel speckle noise reduction technique *History Compounding* is invented. Afterwards, the detection of the critical cochlear endosteum in the improved OCT scans is proposed. Finally, the online planning of the laser ablation is performed according to the resulting residual bone thickness profile above the endosteum.

5.1 Correction of Artefacts in OCT Scans

Similar to other medical imaging systems, OCT suffers from diverse artefacts. We take the OCT scan of the wedge-shaped bone specimen in the feasibility study (figure 3.9b) as an example and plot it here again in figure 5.1a.

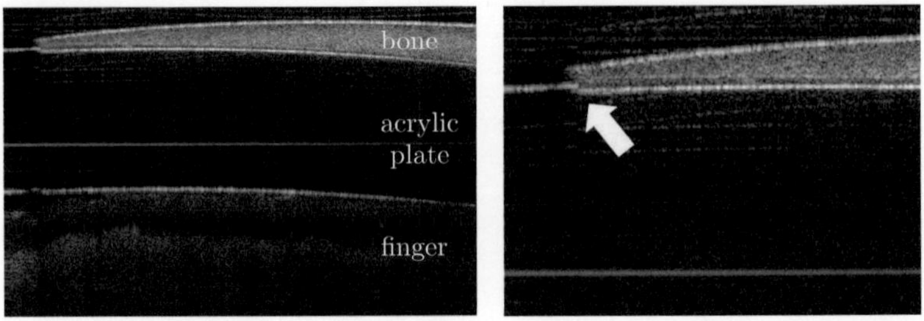

(a) (b)

Figure 5.1: (a) An OCT image with diverse artefacts (the same scan shown in figure 3.9), where the originally planar surfaces are curved and a horizontal stripe can be observed inside the transparent acrylic plate. (b) The magnified view of the top left corner, where the surface of the acrylic plate is shown discontinuous beneath the tip of the bone specimen (arrow).

The following artefacts can be observed from this scan:

- Stripe noises: a horizontal stripe can be clearly seen in the middle of the image inside the acrylic plate. However, the transparent acrylic plate is homogeneous and does not contain any internal structures, which indicates that the stripe is an artefact.
- Curved surfaces: the wedge-shaped bone specimen and acrylic plate have originally planar surfaces, which are however shown curved instead of straight lines in the OCT scans.
- Discontinuous surface: the flat surface of the acrylic plate seems to have a stair-shaped structure under the tip of the bone specimen, as marked in figure 5.1b.

Obviously, it is impossible to correctly detect the position and shape of the critical structure without correction of the artefacts in advance. In the following, methods of correcting these three kinds of artefacts will be developed one by one.

5.1.1 Suppression of Stripe Noises

5.1.1.1 Mechanism

Although the stripe noise can be easily distinguished from the acrylic plate in the example of figure 5.1a, it will be difficult to recognize if the stripe is partly hidden in other structures. Figure 5.2 shows two examples containing relatively weak horizontal stripes, which may not be immediately noticed at first view. In addition to the horizontal ones, bright vertical stripe noises can be observed in figure 5.2b. In the following, the reasons of the stripes are first analysed.

Horizontal Stripe Noise The horizontal stripe is caused by inaccurately acquired background. Reviewing the workflow of OCT A-scan reconstruction (section 3.1.5), background noises are acquired without sample during system calibration and subtracted from each A-scan acquired later. However, certain wavelengths in the sweeping range of the OCT light source are strongly absorbed by water molecules floating in the air, giving sharp absorption lines in the acquired spectra of the background, which occur periodically due to the periodic sweeping through the wavelength band.

For all A-scans acquired after the calibration, the subtraction of the background spectra with periodic sharp absorption lines will result in periodic sharp lines with high amplitudes in the acquired spectra accordingly. These lines lead to high magnitudes at the corresponding spectral components after the Fourier transform, resulting in brighter pixels in the A-scan at these positions. Moreover, the same background is subtracted from each A-scan, so that brighter pixels always occur at the same positions in all A-scans, leading to the horizontal stripes crossing over the whole image. In the case of a three-dimensional OCT volume, the brighter voxels will build up a horizontal lamellar-shaped noisy layer in the 3D space accordingly.

Vertical Stripe Noise The vertical stripe is a similar phenomenon to the *specular highlight*, which is the result of specular reflection and a common phenomenon in medical optical instruments [AGAL10]. It happens when the target tissue surface is glossy and its normal is exactly the bisector between the incoming light and the direction of the viewer (e.g. camera), so that all of the incident light is reflected to the camera and results in saturated white in the acquired images.

In the case of the OCT, the optical path from the light source and back to the detector is the same. Therefore, if the local sample surface is glossy and perpendicular to the incident beam, specular reflection will happen. Having the same phase as each other, interference occurs between the incoming and reflected light that saturates the photodiodes of the detector. These saturations give sharp edges in the spectra of the involved A-scans, attributing to all spectral components after the Fourier transform. The complete A-scan shows therefore saturated white in the reconstructed OCT image, which are exactly the reason for the bright vertical stripes.

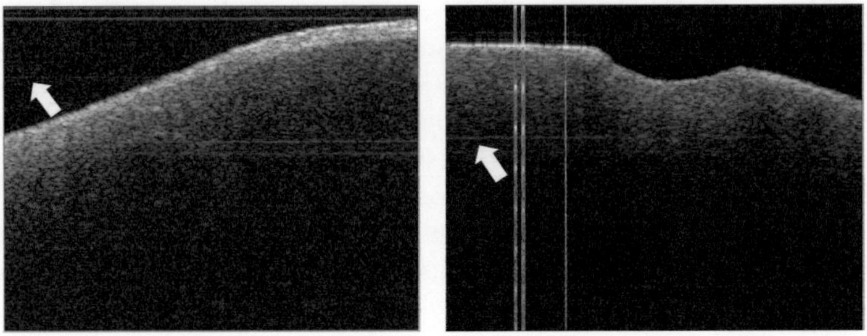

(a) (b)

Figure 5.2: (a-b) OCT images of fresh porcine cochlea polluted by stripe noises: (a) Two groups of double stripes can be observed at the top and in the middle part of the image. Another weaker single stripe (arrow) exists between the two double stripes; (b) Strong vertical stripe noises and a weak horizontal stripe (arrow) can be observed.

5.1.1.2 Stripe Noise Detection

Horizontal Stripe Noise The basic idea of detecting the horizontal stripe noises is quite simple, that is, the bright straight lines crossing over the whole image (or a planar lamellar-shaped layer in three-dimensional case) are impossible to be natural anatomical structures in the lateral skull base. The noisy lines can hence be detected by recognizing the special horizontal structures.

The most intuitive characteristic of the straight noisy lines is that they are brighter than the neighbouring lines. Observing the stripe noises in figure 5.2a more closely, it can be further discovered that the stripe noises have overridden the salt-and-pepper noises locally, so that the values of the pixels within the noisy lines are more homogeneous than their neighbours. Considering these two characteristics, it can be derived that the horizontal sum of the i-th line $s(i)$ should be the local maximum and the intra-line standard deviation $\sigma(i)$ should be local minimum at the axial position of horizontal stripe noises.

Figure 5.3a and b show the s- and σ-profile of the OCT image in figure 5.2a respectively, where the lines in the original OCT image are numbered from the top to the bottom with increasing line ID. In the s-profile, two double peaks can be clearly seen at the positions of line 1-30 and line 160-190, which are corresponding to the two groups of double stripes in the original scan. However, the single stripe near the line 85 cannot be clearly distinguished from figure 5.3a due to the low intensity of the stripe noise, although a small peak may also be observed at this position. On the other hand, the σ-profile shows clear grooves at the single stripe near line 85 and the double stripes at line 160-190. Due to the fact that no structures but salt-and-pepper noises can be measured in air, the intra-line standard deviation is small for all lines at the top of the image, so that the grooves of the double stripes at the line 1-30 can not be distinguished from the neighbouring lines.

For a robust detection of the horizontal stripes, the s and σ-profiles have to be considered simultaneously. The reciprocal $1/\sigma$ of the σ-profile is calculated in order to transform the grooves into peaks and then multiplied with the s-profile, so that the peaks from both profiles will be emphasised. The resulting profile of s/σ has hence clear peaks at the position of the stripe noises (figure 5.3c). Moreover, near the line 50 in the original OCT image, the surface slope turns to be quasi horizontal so that a small peak and a shallow groove can be observed in s- and σ-profile respectively. It is difficult to determine, whether there is a noisy line at this axial position or not. From the s/σ-profile however, it can be uniquely determined that no stripe noise exists there due to the low s/σ value and can be removed by simple thresholding using the average value of the whole profile.

The peaks in the s/σ-profile can be considered as typical discontinuities of a time domain signal, while wavelet is sensible for such sudden changes of the signal amplitude [Liu05]. Therefore, the continuous wavelet transform (CWT) of the s/σ-profile is calculated in order to determine the exact position of the peaks. Considering the shape of the peaks, the Mexican Hat mother wavelet having a similar form as the peaks is chosen. Further observation reveals that the horizontal stripe noises have typically a width of 4-6 pixels, which correspond to the Mexican Hat wavelet with the scale of 1-2. The resulting wavelet coefficients have therefore relatively larger values at the position of the peaks. Once again, multiplication is applied to the wavelet coefficients calculated with the scale 1 and 2 to emphasis the peaks and the result is shown in figure 5.3d, in which five peak positions corresponding to the two double stripes and one single stripe in the original scan can be uniquely identified. The actual widths of the stripes can then be easily measured from the peaks in figure 5.3c.

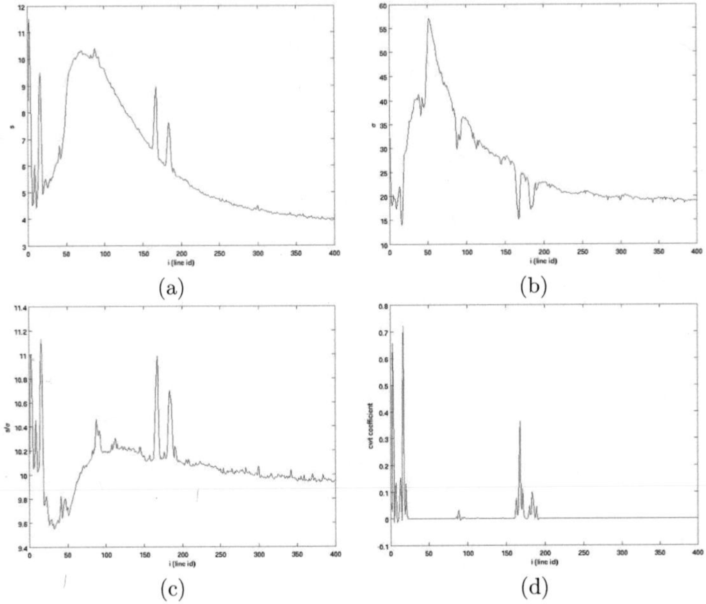

Figure 5.3: Evaluation of single horizontal lines in figure 5.2a, where line ID 1-400 correspond to the horizontal lines from top to bottom: (a) Profile of $s(i)$, which is the sum of all pixels in the i-th line. (b) Profile of $\sigma(i)$, which is the intra-line standard deviation of pixels in the i-th line. (c) The profile of the quotient s/σ. (d) The product of wavelet coefficients of s/σ using Mexican Hat mother wavelet with the scale 1 and 2.

The above procedure is also capable for a three-dimensional OCT volume. Instead of detecting the noises in each single frame, several frames are chosen and concatenated one after another in the horizontal direction, resulting in an extended frame with the size of $h \times kw$, where h and w are the height and width of the original single frame and k is the number of chosen frames. The above procedure is then applied to the extended frame, which will make the detection more robust.

In some cases, stripe noise might be hidden in the anatomical structures in single frames, but it is unlikely to be hidden in all frames of the volume and hence detectable in the extended frame. Moreover, some non-lamellar-shaped anatomical structures might be shown as a quasi horizontal line crossing over a single frame, which will however appear at different axial positions in the extended frame. The structure will therefore not be recognized as a horizontal stripe noise. Empirical results reveal that ten to twenty equidistantly distributed frames in a three-dimensional volume are enough for a robust noise detection.

Vertical Stripe Noise As analysed in section 5.1.1.1, the columns with vertical stripe noises have saturated white pixels. The vertical sums of the these columns are hence much higher than the average level of the whole image (figure 5.4a). If such columns exist in an OCT image or volume, due to the significant difference of energy levels as well as the amount of polluted and unpolluted columns, the histogram of the vertical sums of each single column will have a high peak at the lower and sparsely distributed data points in the higher parts (figure 5.4b). A threshold is set at the foot of the peak where the slope of the histogram is nearly horizontal and the vertical stripe noises are then detected by simple thresholding.

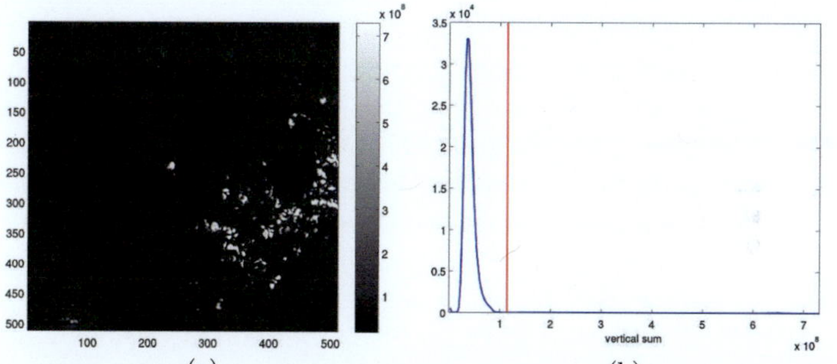

(a) (b)

Figure 5.4: (a) Vertical sum of the columns in an OCT volume with 512 × 512 A-scans where the polluted columns (light gray) can be easily recognized from the unpolluted ones. (b) The histogram of the vertical sums in the Volume, where a threshold is set to the right foot of the peak.

5.1.1.3 Stripe Noises Suppression

Horizontal Stripe Noise The mechanism of the horizontal stripe noises indicates that extra energies are added to the involved lines due to the inaccurately acquired background, which results in the bright stripes. Obviously, these energies have to be subtracted from the involved lines in order to suppress the noises. However, it is impossible to recover the exact value of these energies from the acquired OCT scan itself.

Nevertheless, it can be concluded from figure 5.3a that the s-profile of an OCT scan would be smooth if the horizontal stripe noises did not exist. Therefore, knowing the positions of the lines polluted by the stripe noises, the average energy level in these lines without the pollution of noises can be estimated by linearly interpolating the energy levels of the surrounding lines. Subtracting the difference between the estimated and actual energy level from the involved lines, the horizontal stripe noises can be suppressed.

The effect of this approach is shown in figure 5.5a and b, where the horizontal stripe noises in the images are macroscopically eliminated. It should be noticed that the suppression is based on the estimation of the energy level, which is not an accurate approach. As a result, if we observe the image more closely, traces of the horizontal stripe noises are still visible. Nevertheless, the remaining traces are so slight that they will no more be mistaken for any internal structures of the sample.

Vertical Stripe Noise Unlike the horizontal stripe noises which bring extra energy to the involved lines, the strong interference caused by specular reflection leads to saturated highlighted pixels that flush all usable information in the involved columns (figure 5.2b). In the field of conventional camera systems, which also suffer from the same phenomenon, one of the common methods of inpainting the specular highlights is retrieving the damaged pixels from a series of frames of a video [VPH+02, Kok04, TFMY12]. This method is obviously not feasible for the inpainting of a single OCT scan. Alternatively, a visually pleasing inpainting may also be achieved by calculating weighted sum [CLT+07, OHL+07, AGAL10] or diffusion [PLQS03, BSV13] of the surrounding undamaged pixels in a single image.

In the case of the vertical stripe noises flushing the columns from top to bottom completely, valid pixels are only available in the horizontal direction. Therefore, the simplest inpainting strategy is horizontal linear interpolation of the pixels in the first valid columns on both sides of the detected vertical stripe noises. Figure 5.5b shows the effect of inpainting the OCT scan from figure 5.2b, where the bright vertical stripes are macroscopically removed. Similar as the case of horizontal stripe noise suppression, slight traces of the stripe noises are still visible in the resulting image.

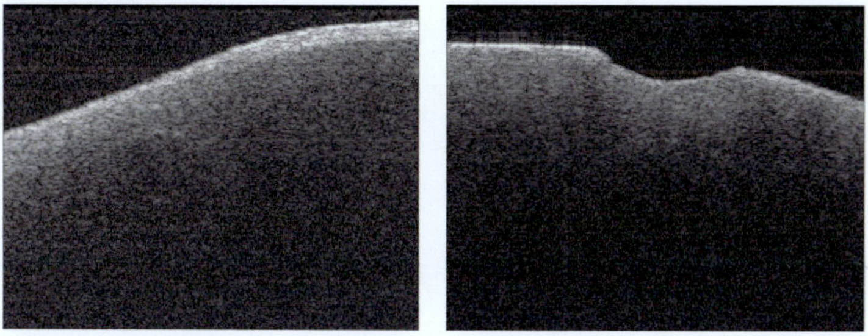

(a) (b)

Figure 5.5: (a-b) Effect of stripe noise suppression. The original OCT scans are shown in figure 5.2a-b.

Remark 5.1. One should be aware that the above approach for suppression of vertical stripe noise only generates the visually pleasing images. It does not recover any usable information about the internal structures in the involved lines. Therefore, the positions of the detected specular reflections are saved and the involved columns are ignored for the segmentation in section 5.3.

5.1.2 Fan Distortion Correction

5.1.2.1 Mechanism

In order to generate three-dimensional scans of the sample, most OCT systems are equipped with scanning optics (refer to section 3.1.1) to deflect the measuring beam on a two-dimensional scan field. The scanners lead to an artefact so called *fan distortion*, which is the reason for the curved surfaces observed in figure 5.1.

Figure 5.6a illustrates the internal structure of a double galvanometric scanner consisting of two perpendicular scanning mirrors and a focusing lens. Obviously, it is physically impossible to locate the focal point O of the lens simultaneously on both of the two mirror centres. In order to prevent the situation that one of the two mirrors is located too far from the focal point, the scanning optics is commonly constructed such that

O is located between the two mirrors. Without loss of generality, assume the distance between one of the two mirror centres O' and the lens is s; the focal length of the lens is f, as illustrated in figure 5.6b. All outgoing beams will be focused to a point located at s' on the optical axis, where s' can be calculated according to the following **lens equation** [DiM12]:

$$\frac{1}{s} + \frac{1}{s'} = \frac{1}{f} \tag{5.1}$$

It can easily be derived that

$$\begin{cases} s' = \infty, & \text{when s=f} \quad (5.2a) \\ s' > 0, & \text{when s>f} \quad (5.2b) \\ s' < 0, & \text{when s<f} \quad (5.2c) \end{cases}$$

Consequently, the outgoing beam vectors $\vec{BC}$ and $\vec{AD}$ will intersect at an infinite point and hence be parallel to the optical axis of the lens for the case (5.2a), so that $|AB| = |CD|$, where $|\cdot|$ denotes the length of the line segment. For the case (5.2b), $\vec{BC'}$ and $\vec{AD'}$ will intersect at a finite distance s' on the right side of the lens, so that $|C'D'| < |CD| = |AB|$ in figure 5.6b. Similarly, $\vec{BC'}$ and $\vec{AD'}$ will intersect backwards at the finite distance s' on the left side of the lens for the case (5.2c), so that $|C'D'| > |AB|$.

Therefore, the A-scans of the OCT are actually not parallel to each other for these two cases. Moreover, the path length along different optical paths are also different, for example the path $|O'EF| \neq |O'BC'|$, so that the points with a same distance to the OCT detector are located on a curved surface rather than on a plane. As a result, the acquired volumes are fan-shaped instead of rectangular (figure 5.6c).

However, while reconstructing two-dimensional and three-dimensional images, no special treatment has been taken to compensate the above effects and all A-scans are regarded to be acquired from a rectangular region (figure 3.2), which leads to the distortion in the OCT images. Depending on the positional relationship between the focal point and the mirror centre, the fan distortion will have two different shapes, so that the originally straight line in the region will be bent either upwards or downwards, as illustrated in figure 5.6d.

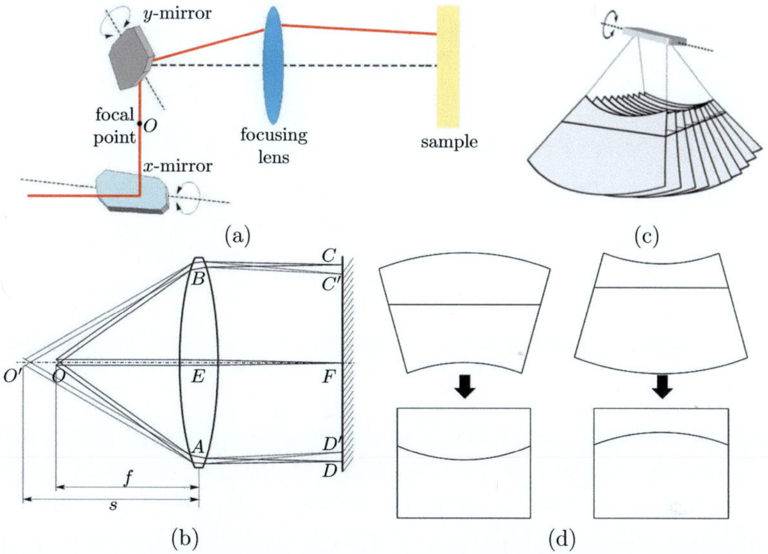

Figure 5.6: (a) A two-dimensional galvanometric scanner with the lens focal point O located between the two mirrors [OSG+10]. (b) Beam deflections after being refracted by a thin lens [OSRM09]. (c) The acquired OCT volume is actually not rectangular but fan-shaped [dJBB+13]. (d) Different shapes of fan distortion in the case of (left) x-mirror with $s > f$ and (right) y-mirror with $s < f$.

5.1.2.2 Correction of Fan Distortion

The procedure of displaying a fan-shaped region as rectangular one (figure 5.6d) can be divided into two steps: first, translate each acquired A-scan along its original direction and align their lower ends to a straight base line. Then tilt the A-scans so that they are perpendicular to the base line and adjust the distance between the A-scans to be equidistant, as illustrated in figure 5.7.

In many cases, the tilting-angles of the A-scans are so small that the tilting and distance adjustment in figure 5.7c have very little influence on the distortion in comparison to the translation. For the sake of simplicity, the influence of the tilting is neglected in the following correction.

In order to measure the translations of the A-scans, the surface of an aluminium plate was chosen as calibration plane. An OCT scan of the whole scan field centred at the mirror position $(0, 0)$ was acquired. Due to the fact that the translation is constant in each A-scan, the calibration plane can be placed arbitrarily within the imaging range and does not necessarily have to be perpendicular to the optical axis of the OCT.

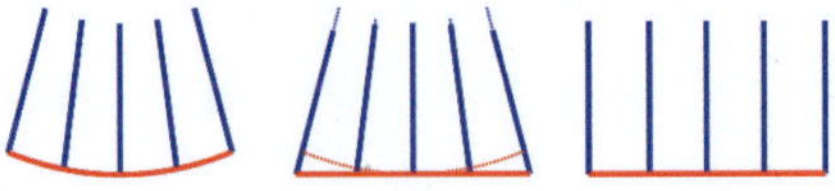

Figure 5.7: The procedure of displaying a fan-shaped region as rectangular one. (a) The original A-scans acquired in a fan-shaped region. (b) Align the A-scans to a base line. (c) Tilt the aligned A-scans to be perpendicular to the base line and adjust the distance to make them equidistant.

Figure 5.8a and b show two OCT scans acquired in the scan directions of the x- and y-mirrors respectively. In both directions, the planar surface is bent for about 100-140 μm over the whole span of 10 mm. Noticing that the focal point of the lens is located between the two mirrors (figure 5.6a) with $s > f$ for the x-mirror and $s < f$ for the y-mirror, the surface is hence bent to the opposite direction in the scans.

With simple thresholding, the distorted three-dimensional surface profile of the calibration plane can be reconstructed (figure 5.8c) and a bi-cubic B-spline surface fitting (refer to [PBP02]) is applied to it. Considering that the calibration plane is not perfectly perpendicular to the optical axis of the OCT, the normal of the calibration plane is retrieved from the four corners of the resulting spline surface. Compensating the slope of the plane and normalizing the compensated spline surface to the mirror position $(0, 0)$ (centre point of the scan field), the profile of A-scan translation over the whole scan field purely due to the fan distortion can be obtained. Its negative profile $p(x, y)$ is exactly the correction profile for the fan distortion, which has a saddle-shaped form (figure 3.9d).

Consequently, for any A-scan acquired at a given mirror position (x, y), simply translate the whole A-scan upwards for $p(x, y)$ pixels and the fan distortion can be corrected. In the case of non-integer $p(x, y)$, the values of pixels are calculated by linear interpolation of neighbouring pixels above and below the new axial position after the translation. Applying this correction to the curved surface profile in figure 5.8c and the B-scan in figure 3.9, the fan distortion is perfectly corrected in both examples, where the originally planar surfaces are now shown as straight lines (figure 5.8e and f).

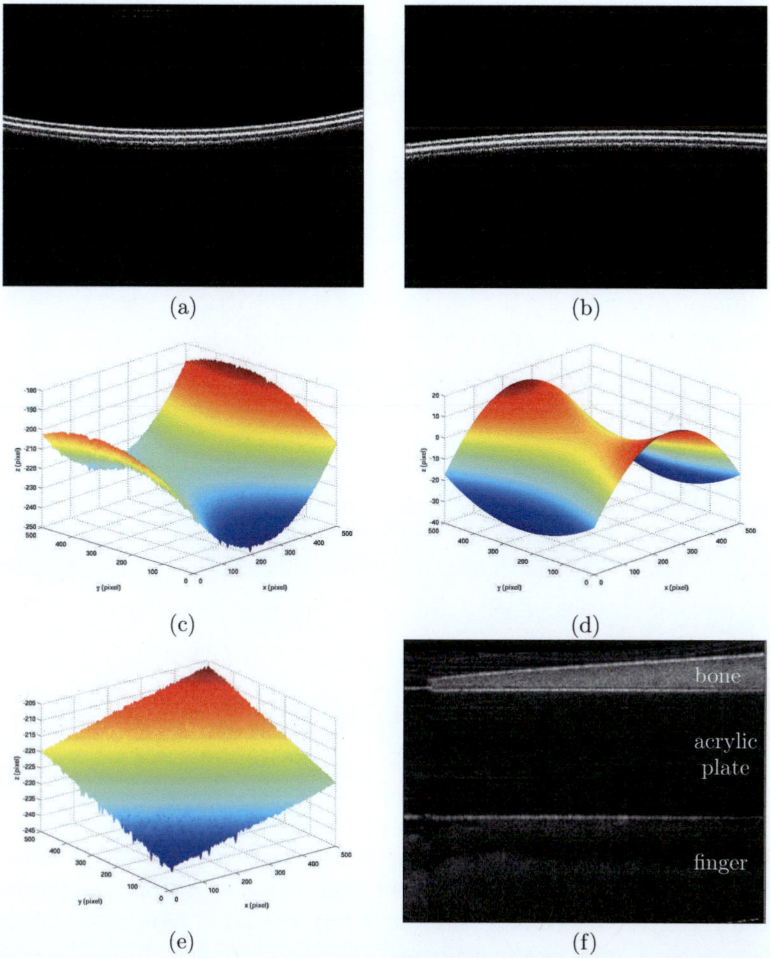

Figure 5.8: (a-b) OCT scans of a planar calibration plane (aluminium plate) acquired in the scan directions of (a) x-mirror and (b) y-mirror. (c) Reconstructed 3D surface profile of the calibration plane. (d) Correction profile $p(x, y)$ for the fan-distortion obtained by B-spline surface fitting. (e-f) Results of the fan distortion correction: (e) the calibration plane and (f) a wedge-shaped bone specimen with acrylic plate and finger underneath (original curved scan see figure 3.9b).

Remark 5.2. The above bi-cubic B-spline fitting based approach provides a simple but effective solution to the correction of fan distortion. Compared with correction methodologies of other authors, no complicated modelling of the scanning optics [WRRI02, dJBB+13] and special system configuration [OSRM09, WLS+13] are required.

However, it should be noticed that the approach has neglected the influence of the small angle[1] of A-scan tilting and non-equidistant A-scan distribution (figure 5.7c), which excludes the application of this approach for severe distorted scanning optics with extremely large scan field. Nevertheless, the results in figure 5.8 indicate that the accuracy is already sufficient for the correction of a $10 \times 10\,\text{mm}^2$ region, which is the typical scan field size of most commercial OCT systems.

For the case of laser-cochleostomy, a scan region with the size of only about $2 \times 2\,\text{mm}^2$ in the centre of the scan field is required. Within this region, the fan distortion is much slighter (see figure 5.8d), so that the above calibration method is already accurate enough. Moreover, the registration method proposed later in section 6.3 creates a point-wise mapping between the distorted OCT volume and the working space of the CO_2 laser. The inaccuracy induced by neglecting the A-scan tilting and non-equidistant distribution will hence not influence the precision of the ablation.

5.1.3 Refractive Index Compensation

5.1.3.1 Mechanism

The third artefact observed in the figure 5.1b is the result of uncompensated speed of light in different materials. Recalling the working principle of OCT (section 3.1.1 and 3.1.2), the OCT interprets the time delay of the echoes as the depth where the echoes come from. However, OCT does not take the different speeds of light variations in different media into account. As a result, an echo that comes back at the time point t will be displayed at the depth of $c \cdot t/2$ no matter where it comes from. Here c is the speed of light in vacuum and the factor 2 denotes the path back and forth between the OCT and the structure.

[1] Figure 5.8a-c seem to have large angular distortion, which is visual illusion due to non-equal coordinates in xy and z directions by plotting. As mentioned in main text, the z value changes only for 100-140 μm over a scan range of $10 \times 10\,\text{mm}^2$, which is still quite "flat".

Specifically for the example in figure 5.1b, suppose the distance from the bone surface to the OCT device is D and the bone thickness at the specimen tip is d, as illustrated in figure 5.9a. For the sake of simplicity, the velocity of light propagation in the relatively homogeneous compact bone tissue of cochlea is assumed to be constant. Observe two points P_1 and P_2 on the acrylic plate surface, where P_1 is exposed to the air directly while P_2 is located beneath the tip of the bone specimen. It can then be easily derived that P_1 and P_2 will be displayed at the axial positions z_1 and z_2 with

$$\begin{cases} z_1 = c \cdot (D/\nu_{\text{a}} + d/\nu_{\text{a}}) \\ z_2 = c \cdot (D/\nu_{\text{a}} + d/\nu_{\text{b}}) \end{cases} \tag{5.3}$$

where ν_{a} and ν_{b} are the speeds of light in air and compact bone tissue respectively. According to [YY97, DiM12], it is always helpful in optics to use the refractive index defined by equation (2.4) instead of using the speed of light directly. Then the equation (5.3) can be rewritten as

$$\begin{cases} z_1 = n_{\text{a}} D + n_{\text{a}} d \\ z_2 = n_{\text{a}} D + n_{\text{b}} d \end{cases} \tag{5.4}$$

where n_{a} and n_{b} are the refractive indices of air and compact bone tissue respectively. For more general situations, suppose the incident beam has penetrated through k layers of media with the refractive indices n_i and the thickness d_i before reaching a structure of interest. Then the structure will be displayed at the axial position

$$z = \sum_{i=1}^{k} n_i d_i \tag{5.5}$$

In most situations, the speed of light in any medium is slower than in vacuum, so that $n > 1$ always applies[2], while the refractive index of air $n_{\text{a}} = 1.00029$ is often regarded as 1 in the practice [HZ02]. It can hence be derived from equation (5.4) that $z_1 = D + d$ and $z_2 = D + n_{\text{b}} d$ with $n_{\text{b}} > 1$, so that $z_1 < z_2$. This means that the point P_2 will be shown at a deeper position than the point P_1 in the acquired OCT image (figure 5.9b), which is exactly the artefact observed in figure 5.1b.

[2] An exception is the X-radiation, which is however irrelevant in our case, details see [HZ02].

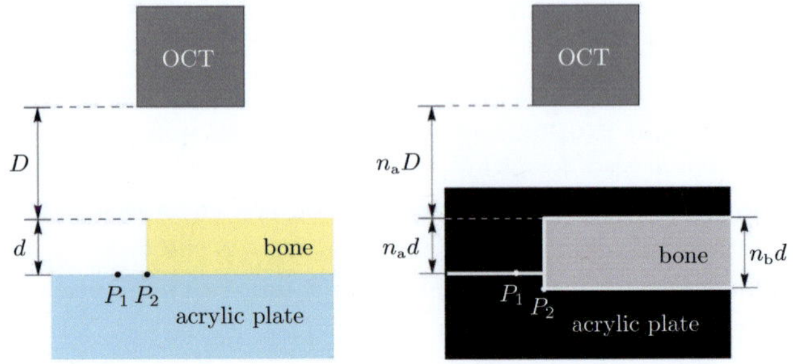

(a) (b)

Figure 5.9: (a) Schematic diagram of the experimental setup used for the acquisition of the image in figure 5.1b. (b) Due to the different refractive indices of air n_a and compact bone tissue n_b, the originally coplanar points P_1 and P_2 are shown at different axial positions in the acquired OCT image (the black rectangular region).

Particularly, the **optical path length** from point A to B is defined as

$$\text{OPL}_A^B = \int_A^B n dl \tag{5.6}$$

where l is the physical path length of the light travelled in the real world. Moreover, if the refractive index along the physical path AB is piecewise constant, then the equation (5.6) can be written in the discrete form

$$\text{OPL}_A^B = \sum_m n_m l_m \tag{5.7}$$

Notice that the equation (5.5) has exactly the same form as equation (5.7). Therefore, the axial position z in OCT images actually correspond to the optical path length between the structure of interest to the OCT device, not the physical path length. The resulting distortion of the image can be hence quantitatively described by the difference between the optical and physical path length as

$$\begin{aligned} \Delta l &= \sum_{i=1}^{k} n_i d_i - \sum_{i=1}^{k} d_i \\ &= \sum_{i=1}^{k} (n_i - 1) d_i \end{aligned} \tag{5.8}$$

From equation (5.8), it can be further deduced that the distortion Δl caused by a medium with a refractive index $n > 1$ is proportional to its thickness. This explains the discontinuous cochlear endosteum observed in figure 3.8a, where the discontinuous thickness distribution of overlaying bone tissue within the laser ablated crater results in a discontinuity of the distortion Δl, which makes the structure to be displayed irregular.

5.1.3.2 Algorithm of Refractive Index Compensation

In order to correct the distortion due to the different optical and physical path lengths, the influence of every medium layer between the structure of interest and the OCT has to be compensated. For the case of laser-cochleostomy, the measuring beam of the OCT will first penetrate the air and then the bony shell of the cochlea before it reaches the bone-endosteum-perilymph interface.

As mentioned above, the refractive index of air n_a can be regarded as 1, so that the distortion caused by the air layer is zero according to equation (5.8). Therefore, the bone layer is the only source of the distortion in our case. In other words, the OCT image is not distorted from the top until reaching the bone surface and a correction of distortion is only necessary for the pixels underneath.

Supposing that the bone surface intersects an A-scan at the point S and observe an arbitrary point P in the same A-scan beneath S. If the physical path length from S to P is δ, then the optical path length from the S to P is

$$\mathrm{OPL}_S^P(\delta) = n_b \delta \tag{5.9}$$

which indicates that the line segment SP will be stretched for the factor n_b in the acquired OCT image. Hence, a trivial idea of the distortion correction is to compensate the refractive index n_b and compress the stretched line segment SP back to its original length δ. However, if n_b is a non-integer, the pixels will also be located at non-integer positions after the compression and thus cannot be displayed as an image.

Therefore, instead of compressing the distorted OCT A-scan, the to be calculated distortion-free A-scans are stretched by the factor of n_b, overlaid to the distorted ones. Each pixel is then calculated by linearly interpolating the neighbouring distorted pixels, as described in algorithm 5.1. The input A-scan is assumed to have n pixels.

Algorithm 5.1: Compensation of Refractive Index n_b

Input: Distorted A-scan $I_{n\times 1}$
Output: Distortion-free A-scan $I'_{n\times 1}$
Determine the axial position z_S of the surface point S
for $i \leftarrow 1$ **to** n **do** `// for each pixel` P `in` I'
  if $i < z_S$ **then** `// pixel above the surface`
    $I'_i \leftarrow I_i$ `// no distortion, copy the pixel`
  else
    $j \leftarrow z_S + (i - z_S) \cdot n_b$ `// stretch physical path` SP
    if $j > n$ **then** `//` j `exceeds lower image boundary`
      $I'_i \leftarrow 0$
    else `// linear interpolate the neighbours`
      $\alpha \leftarrow j - \text{floor}(j)$
      $I'_i \leftarrow \alpha \cdot I_{\text{ceil}(j)} + (1-\alpha) \cdot I_{\text{floor}(j)}$

However, two very important parameters necessary for algorithm 5.1 are still unknown, namely the axial position of the surface z_S and the refractive index of compact bone tissue n_b. These two parameters will be determined in the next two sections.

5.1.3.3 Sample Surface Detection

Analysis of Edge Property As described in section 2.2.1, when the light enters one medium from another one, reflection happens on the interface between the two media. For small incident angles, the ratio of the reflected energy to the incident energy can be described by equation (2.6). Considering the case of OCT, only the fraction of the incident light that comes back exactly along the original optical path of the incident light can reach the detector (figures 3.3-3.5), so that the condition of small incident angle is always satisfied for the measured echo.

Denoting the ratio between the refractive indices of the two media by $\eta = n_2/n_1 > 0$ and the reflectance by γ, then the equation (2.6) can be rewritten as a function of $\gamma(\eta)$:

$$\gamma(\eta) = \frac{I_r}{I_i} = \left|\frac{\eta - 1}{\eta + 1}\right|^2 \tag{5.10}$$

It can easily be inferred that $\gamma(\eta) = 0$ if and only if $\eta = 1 \Leftrightarrow n_2 = n_1$. Therefore, no light will be reflected inside a homogeneous medium, for example the air and acrylic plate, which are hence always dark in the OCT images. Contrarily, as long as the medium is slightly inhomogeneous so that $\eta \neq 1 \Rightarrow \gamma(\eta) \neq 0$, the measuring beam will be reflected at the inhomogeneity inside the medium itself and not necessarily only at the interface to another medium. This is the reason why the pixels inside the bone tissue are also bright in the example OCT scans shown in previous sections. From equation (5.10) can further be derived that

$$\gamma'(\eta) \begin{cases} > 0, \text{ when } \eta > 1 \\ = 0, \text{ when } \eta = 1 \\ < 0, \text{ when } 0 < \eta < 1 \end{cases} \tag{5.11}$$

Equation (5.11) indicates that γ reaches a global minimum when $\eta = 1$; increases monotonically for $\eta > 1$ and decreases monotonically for $0 < \eta < 1$, as shown in figure 5.10a. Notice that when $n_2 > n_1$, $\eta = n_2/n_1$ is greater than 1 and increases with the increasing difference between n_1 and n_2; when $n_2 < n_1$, $\eta = n_2/n_1$ is less than 1 and decreases with the increasing difference between n_1 and n_2. In other words, the larger is the difference between the refractive indices of the two media, the larger is the reflectance, resulting in more reflected fraction of the incident light and hence stronger echo.

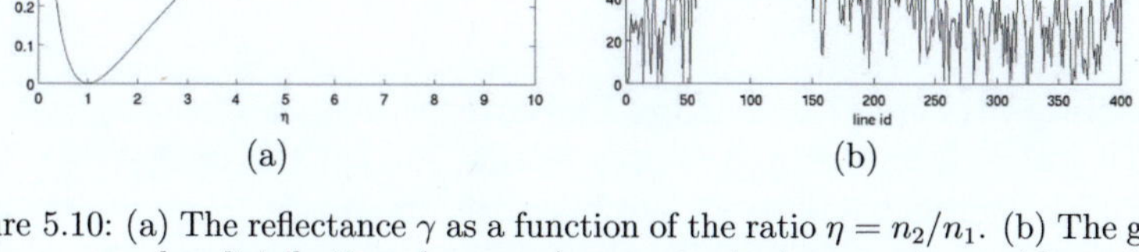

(a) (b)

Figure 5.10: (a) The reflectance γ as a function of the ratio $\eta = n_2/n_1$. (b) The gray value distribution along an A-scan acquired on porcine cochlea, where a very clear jump can be observed at the air-bone interface.

Obviously, the difference of refractive indices between air and tissue sample is much larger than the difference due to inhomogeneity inside the biological tissue of the same kind. Therefore, the intensity of the echo from the most superficial air-tissue interface is always stronger than that from the tissue layers underneath. Moreover, biological tissues are never perfectly homogeneous and diffusing. The intensities of both the incident measuring beam and reflected echo are hence weakened due to scattering into other directions as well as energy absorption in the tissue. Contrarily, the echo from the air-tissue interface has only transmitted through the air and remains unattenuated. Such an effect makes the difference of the echo more significant.

Summarised, no matter what kind of tissue the sample is, the air above the tissue surface will be dark while the air-tissue interface will be the brightest structure of the sample until the next tissue boundary (if there exist any) in the OCT scans. Hence, it is theoretically guaranteed that

Proposition 5.3. *The most superficial air-tissue interface is always an edge-strong boundary in OCT scans.*

Proposition 5.3 explains why all the air-sample boundaries in any example OCT scans shown in previous sections are always high contrast ones. Figure 5.10b shows the gray value distribution along an A-scan acquired on a fresh porcine cochlea, where the interface between the air and bone surface can be immediatly recognized in this single A-scan without observing the whole image. The intensity of pixels beneath the surface then decreases exponentially with the depth.

The detection of the edge-strong air-tissue interface is hence straight forward and divided into two steps: spatial filtering based edge detection in each single frame and global morphological operation based surface smoothing in the whole three dimensional volume. In the following, the OCT scan of the human cochlea in figure 3.6b is taken as example to demonstrate the procedure.

Spatial Filtering Based Edge Detection As most imaging systems, OCT suffers from salt-and-pepper noises, so that the images especially the dark regions are blurred. For instance, the pixels above the air-bone interface in figure 5.10b, which are supposed to be zero according to the above analysis, have however non-zero gray values with oscillation in the range from about 0 to 50. The first step is hence to apply the median filter (refer to section 4.1) to the image, which is particularly effective for suppressing salt-and-pepper noises [GW02]. The size of the filter is chosen according to the noise level in the given OCT scans individually. For the particular example in figure 3.6b, a 5×5 median filter is applied and the resulting image is shown in figure 5.11a. As expected, the noises are suppressed and a sharper boundary is obtained.

The routine procedure for detecting such a clear dark to bright boundary is to apply the Sobel operators defined by equations (4.4) and (4.5) to the image, which calculates the sum of the absolute values of vertical and horizontal gradients. Noticing that the boundary to be detected is a dark to bright one in the vertically downward direction, so that the pixels on the air-tissue boundary must have positive vertical gradient after application of the vertical Sobel operator. Therefore, instead of using equation (4.5) directly, the absolute value of the vertical gradient $|G_{\text{vert}}|$ is replaced by $\max(G_{\text{vert}}, 0)$,[3] so that all negative vertical gradients will be set to zero. Thus, all bright to dark boundaries will be suppressed to a certain degree, no matter a real boundary like the cochlear endosteum (figure 5.11a) or a fake one due to noises. The resulting gradient map is shown in figure 5.11b, in which the air-bone interface is emphasised.

However, the endosteum and non-zero gradients due to noises can still be observed in the gradient map, even in the air above the sample surface. The candidate surface pixels are also not uniquely emphasised, for example a small double-layer structure can be observed in figure 5.11b at the left part of the channel bottom in the cochleostomy. An average filter (equation (4.3) left) with the same size as the previous median filter is hence applied to smooth the obtained gradient map, which diffuses the non-zero gradients isotropically in all directions into the neighbourhood, as shown in figure 5.11c. As expected, the local double-layer structure disappears after the diffusion, so that the surface position can be determined uniquely. Besides, the noises with low intensity above the surface are further weakened while the air-bone interface remains a bright structure with increased thickness compared to figure 5.11b. Considering the convolution-based filtering mechanism defined by equation (4.2), it can be further derived that the thickness of the bright structure is at least the same as the size of the average filter.

The histogram-based thresholding approach used for vertical stripe noise detection (see figure 5.4 and relevant text) is then applied to distinguish candidate boundary pixels from the background. Starting searching from the top of the smoothed gradient map, the position of the diffused

[3] The function $\max(a, b)$ denotes the larger one of a and b.

surface is estimated by locating the first continuous structure in the segmented foreground, which has a thickness larger than the size of the average filter. Notice that the diffusion effect of the average filter is isotropic, the exact position of the interface is therefore the middle curve of the detected wide bright structure. The resulting surface profile is shown in figure 5.11d, which outlines the dark to bright air-bone interface exactly and also matches the manual judgement.

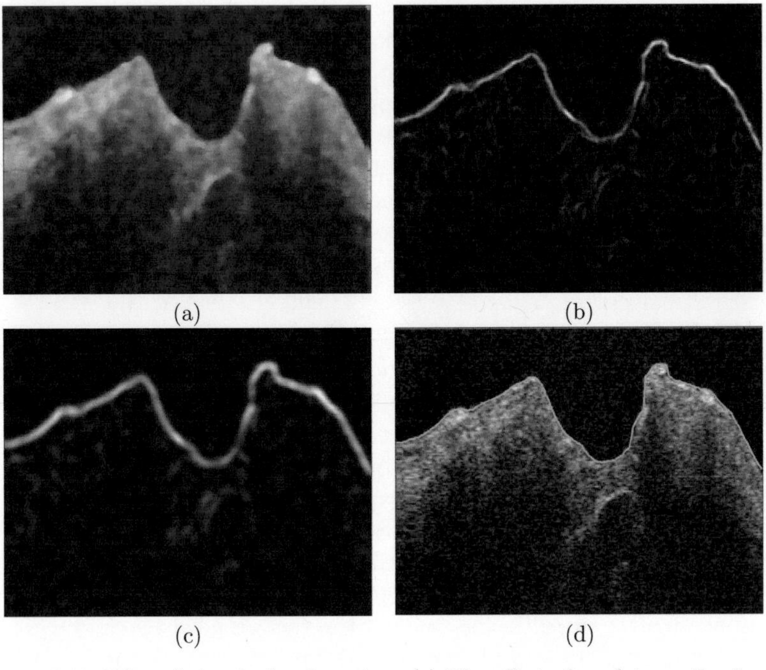

Figure 5.11: Filter chain of edge detection: (a) The effect of applying a 5×5 median filter to figure 3.6b. (b) The corresponding gradient map after the application of Sobel operators. (c) Smoothed gradient map after applying a 5×5 average filter. (d) The air-tissue interface determined by locating the middle curve of the wide bright band in (c).

Applying the above described filter chain to each single frame in the given three-dimensional OCT volume, the 3D-surface profile of the air-sample surface can be obtained preliminarily.

Morphological Operation-Based Surface Smoothing The above proposed filter chain relies on the gray value gradient in a single OCT frame alone without taking the curvature of the extracted surface profile into account. Consequently, the resulting surface profile might deviate from the real boundary in some cases, especially when the input OCT scan has poor image quality. Figure 5.12a shows an example of a slightly curved compact bone specimen with two craters ablated by single laser pulses. The image was acquired by a poorly calibrated OCT, suffering from stronger salt-and-pepper noises and the sample surface looks furry with brush-shaped structures, which actually do not exist at all.

Nevertheless, the preconditions of proposition 5.3 are inherent properties of light and hence always satisfied. As a result, despite the poor image quality, the air-bone interface is still an edge-strong boundary in figure 5.12a. Therefore, it is as usual reasonable to utilize the filter chain above for the surface detection in the poorly acquired OCT image. Considering the higher noise level, the size of median and average filters is set to 9×9 and the resulting surface is plotted in figure 5.12b.

It can be observed that the poor image quality does have negative effects on the edge detection, where the extracted surface follows the fake brush-shaped structures at multiple positions resulting in a deviation of the extracted surface profile. Despite this fact, the macroscopic position of the detected surface is still correct due to the edge-strong property of the air-bone interface and the deviation only occurs locally where the brush-shaped phantoms are significant. Therefore, a post-processing is required to eliminate the local outliers while holding the macroscopic position of the surface profile.

As stated in section 4.3, morphological opening and closing operations are often used for smoothing the contours of an object and hence appropriate tools for this purpose. In order to take advantage of the information in neighbouring frames, the preliminary 3D surface profile obtained from the filter chain is regarded as a two-dimensional gray-scale image. The gray-scale opening and closing operations illustrated in figure 4.6 are performed, where spheres with proper radii are chosen as structuring elements and the sharp peaks and grooves are eliminated after rolling the spheres against the upper- and undersides of the surface to be smoothed. Notice that the noises in the bone tissue beneath the air-bone interface is always stronger than that in the transparent air above, so that the deviation of the surface profile will be mainly downwards with groove-like shape. The gray-scale closing is hence performed first to roll the "rolling ball" from the top and then the opening operation from the underside.

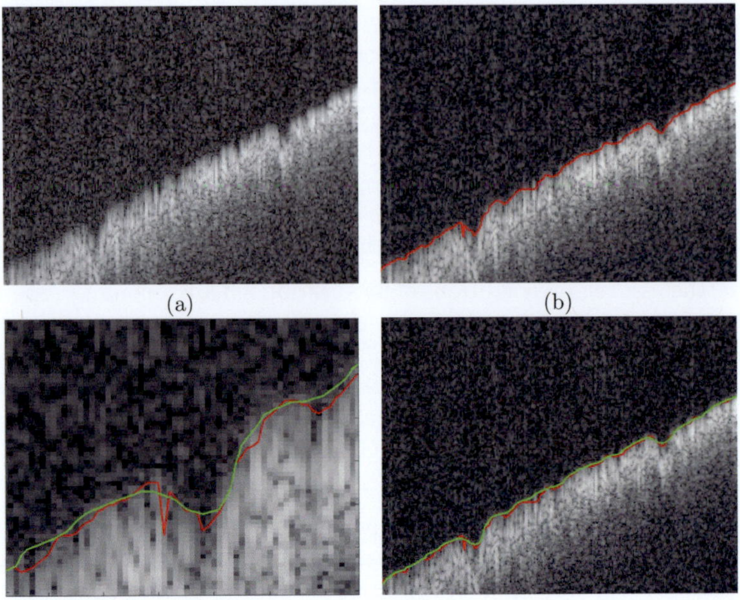

Figure 5.12: (a) An OCT scan acquired by poorly calibrated OCT on a bone specimen with two laser ablated craters located at about the 1/4 and 3/4 of the whole image width in the horizontal direction. (b) The sample surface extracted by the proposed filter chain using 9 × 9 median and average filters. (c-d) Comparison of the extracted surface profile before (red) and after (green) the 3D morphological closing and opening using spheres with radii 5 as structuring elements: (c) the magnified view of the left crater and (d) the whole frame.

As introduced in section 2.1.1, the cochlea consists of dense compact bone tissue without naturally formed porous internal structure. After the removal of the overlaying bone layer, no matter whether done by laser or drill bit, the tiniest structures that may occur on the sample surface during the process of cochleostomy are the craters ablated by single laser pulses seen in figure 5.12a-b. Therefore, the radii of the spherical structuring elements should be chosen a little bit smaller than the craters, so that they can fit into and retain these structures while eliminating other sharper structures that are caused by noises.[4]

[4] If the noise level is so high that the phantom structures have similar size as the craters, the system is completely de-calibrated and an anew calibration or maintenance of the OCT system is mandatory in such a case.

The effect of performing the closing and opening operations using spheres with radius of 5 pixels as structuring element is shown in figure 5.12c-d. From the magnified view it can be observed that the sharp grooves with the width of about 1-3 pixels are successfully eliminated. The overall surface profile in figure 5.12d is smoothed as expected while the two craters are preserved.

Moreover, a quite long segment of the smoothed surface profile (green) near the right lip of the left crater differs from the preliminary profile before smoothing (red), resulting in a more appropriate boundary position. Such a phenomenon is impossible if the morphological operations are performed only within a single frame and demonstrates the effect of the "rolling ball" in 3D, which takes advantage of the information provided by the neighbouring frames. For the OCT volume with normal image quality shown in figure 5.11, no significant change of the surface profile can be observed after applying the morphological operations.

Figure 5.13 shows the final result of applying the complete workflow of the surface detection to an OCT volume of a cochleostomy on a porcine cochlea, where the insertion channel and four tiny laser ablated landmarks (refer to section 6.2 for details) are clearly visible in the obtained surface profile.

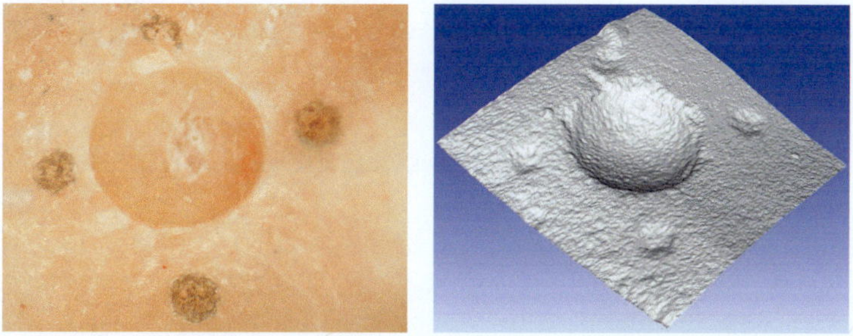

(a) (b)

Figure 5.13: Effect of the complete workflow of sample surface detection: (a) a cochleostomy on a porcine cochlea with four laser ablated landmarks surrounding it under a light microscope; (b) the 3D surface profile extracted from the OCT volume.

Discussion The workflow introduced in this section uses a very simple filter chain and morphological operations instead of using popular high level segmentation techniques such as a deformable model based segmentation or graph based approaches (refer to section 4.2). Although Fuchs et al. [FSK+12] suggested to use an adapted snake for the same purpose (see figure 4.2b), it is here completely unnecessary because the approach was initially designed for detecting edge-weak boundaries and brings no extra benefit in our edge-strong case. Contrarily, applying such a parametric deformable model requires a more complicated parametrization of the weights of the diverse energy terms in the cost function (4.9), which is demanding for the surgeons without background in the field of image segmentation. Considering the low efficiency of the graph based approaches and the high cost for creating training data sets of the active shape models, neither of them are appropriate choices for our case.

Compared to these complicated high-level segmentation techniques, the proposed simple approach takes full advantage of the inherent property of OCT images that the most superficial air-sample interfaces always have high contrast. A robust segmentation reserving the tiniest structure in the input image is achieved, even for the images with very poor image quality like figure 5.12a.

The simple workflow guarantees a high processing efficiency and an intuitive parametrization. The only parameters to be determined by the user are the size of median and average filters as well as the radii of the structuring element for the morphological operations. All these parameters have intuitive geometrical meanings and can be easily determined even by inexperienced users.

5.1.3.4 Determination of Refractive Index

Methodology Having determined the position of the most superficial air-sample interface, the only unknown parameter of algorithm 5.1 is now the refractive index of the bone tissue. Ascenzi et al. [AF59] have determined the refractive index of a single osteone unit, which is the primary anatomical and functional unit of compact bone tissue, to be 1.55-1.56. Some other research groups focus on the refractive indices of diverse components in human teeth. Colston et al. [CJEDS+98] have given an estimation of the refractive indices of enamel to be 1.6 and that of dentin to be 1.5; Meng et al. [MYY+09b] have reported the concrete values of enamel, dentin and cementum are 1.63, 1.54 and 1.58 respectively, while Ohmi et al. [OOYH00] have measured 1.65 for enamel and 1.55 for dentin.

However, the refractive index of cochlea as well as compact bone tissues of other kind have not been provided by any research groups yet. Only a rough estimation could be made from the above values: the refractive indices of bony tissues should be around 1.60. The accurate measurement of the optical properties of biological tissues requires not only special techniques and equipments [CPW90, SKB93], but also corresponding expertise in optical engineering, which are unfortunately unavailable in our research group. A simpler methodology for determination of the refractive index is therefore mandatory.

Reviewing the discussion in section 5.1.3.1 and 5.1.3.2, the bone layer is the only source of the stair-shaped distortion observed at the specimen tip in figure 5.1b, 5.8f and 5.9b. Algorithm 5.1 regards hence the refractive index as the compression factor to compress the bone layer beneath the air-bone interface. It can be easily inferred that if a value smaller or larger than the correct refractive index is applied, the gray part denoting bone tissue in the figure 5.9b will be either insufficiently or over compressed. Only when the correct refractive index is used, the point P_2 could be aligned with P_1 and thus eliminate the distortion.

Based on this consideration, a simple methodology for measuring the refractive index of bone tissue is proposed in algorithm 5.2. The basic idea is to use OCT images distorted due to uncompensated refractive index such as figure 5.1b and 5.8f themselves as calibration images.

Algorithm 5.2: Determination of Refractive Index n_b

Input: Calibration image I
Output: Refractive index n_b

Give a rough estimation of the refractive index n_b
while *distortion is observed in calibration image* I **do**
    Apply algorithm 5.1 to I with current estimation of n_b
    if *insufficient compression* **then**
        increase n_b for Δn
    else if *over compression* **then**
        decrease n_b for Δn

As described above, the initial estimation of n_b for bony tissues could be chosen as 1.60. Considering the axial resolution of 8.41 μm and the 500-800 μm imaging depth of OCT into compact bone tissue (refer to section 3.2.2), only about 100 pixels from the bone surface will be effective to provide the internal information of the sample. Particularly, for the N-th pixel beneath the bone surface, a deviation of ± 0.01 in the estimated n_b will lead to a compression error of

$$\left|\frac{N}{n_b} - \frac{N}{n_b \pm 0.01}\right| = \frac{0.01N}{n_b(n_b \pm 0.01)} \approx \frac{N}{100n_b^2} \tag{5.12}$$

With the refractive index of about 1.60, even the 100th pixel beneath the bone surface will have an error less than half a pixel after the compression. Therefore, an accuracy of two digits after the decimal point is already sufficient for the compression and the Δn in algorithm 5.2 is set to 0.01. Adjusting the value of the refractive index and examining the existence of distortion in the calibration image I manually until the distortion disappears, the accurate value of n_b can be obtained.

Experimental Measurements The methodology above was then experimentally evaluated. Considering that the stair-shaped distortion in figure 5.1b and 5.8f are not significant enough and may make the manual calibration more difficult, a new calibration object with a stair-shaped surface and flat backside was prepared using the CO_2 laser on a fresh bovine compact bone sheet separated from cattle femur with a total thickness of circa 2 mm, as shown in figure 5.14. The stairs were generated by applying a square-shaped ablation pattern on the specimen and each stair has the height of about 140 μm.

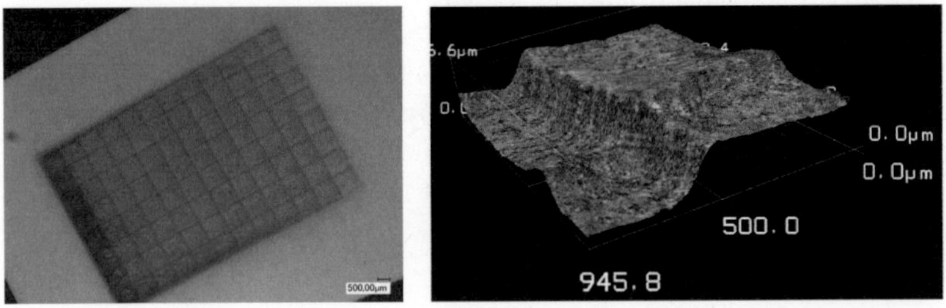

(a) (b)

Figure 5.14: (a) Calibration object (fresh bovine compact bone separated from femur) with stair-shaped surface and flat backside. (b) The 3D surface profile of the stair-shaped structure measured with a laser-scanning microscope (Keyence VK-X200, Keyence Deutschland GmbH, Neu-Isenburg, Germany), where each stair has the height≈140 μm.

OCT scan of the calibration object (figure 5.15a) was performed with a mirror underneath, so that more light can be reflected back from the bone-mirror interface, resulting in stronger echo and much clearer boundary in the calibration scan. Moreover, imaging depth is also significantly increased, where the mirror is still visible with a overlaying bone thickness up to circa 1.5 mm. Thus, a longer and stronger boundary on the backside of the specimen is obtained in the calibration scan, making it much easier for the user to recognize the distortion.

As expected, the varying bone thickness beneath the stairs results in different optical path length to the backside of the specimen, leading the originally flat bone-mirror boundary to be stair-shaped in the calibration scan due to the uncompensated refractive index n_b. Compared to other candidate shapes of calibration object resulting in distortion of other geometric shape, for example circular arc, human eyes are more sensitive to distinguish whether a structure is broken or continuous. Therefore, a more accurate result is expected with the proposed stair-shaped calibration object. By applying algorithm 5.2 to figure 5.15a until the backside forms a perfect straight line again (figure 5.15b), it was determined that the refractive index n_b of bovine compact bone is 1.59.

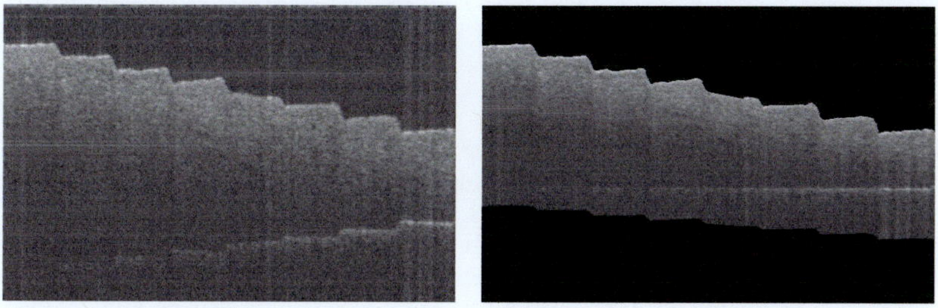

(a) (b)

Figure 5.15: (a) The original OCT scan of the calibration object shown in figure 5.14 with a mirror underneath. (b) Apply algorithm 5.2 until the backside of the specimen to be a straight line again, yielding that $n_b = 1.59$ for bovine compact bone tissue.

In order to examine the correctness of the obtained refractive index, algorithm 5.1 with $n_b = 1.59$ was applied to the distorted OCT scan in figure 5.8f and the result is shown in figure 5.16a. It can be observed that the stair-shaped distortion beneath the specimen tip in figure 5.8f is eliminated and the surface of the acrylic plate is again a straight line after the distortion correction. The application of the procedure to

OCT scans of other stair-shaped specimen with different stair sizes also revealed the same result. This evidence the correctness of the procedure for determination and compensation of the refractive index proposed in algorithms 5.1 and 5.2.

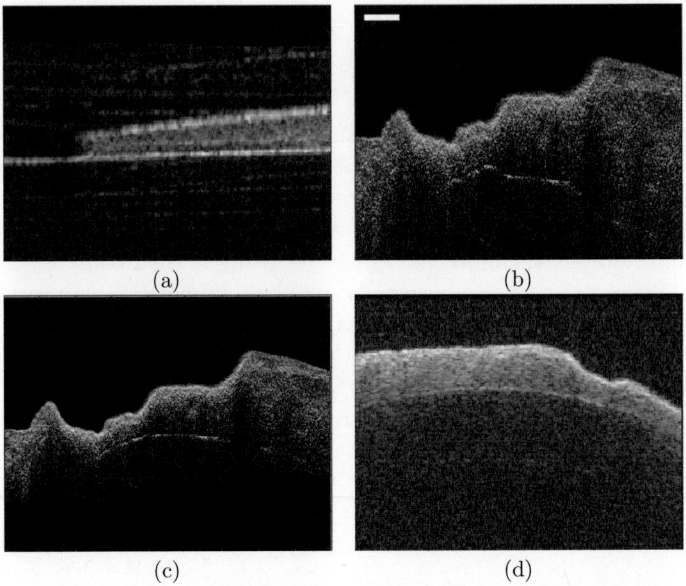

Figure 5.16: (a) The magnified view of the top left part of figure 5.8f after the refractive index compensation using $n_b = 1.59$, where the originally broken acrylic plate surface is now a straight line. (b-c) Determination of the refractive index of cochlea using laser ablated stair-shaped structure: (b) original calibration image, bar=250 μm in air; (c) applying algorithm 5.2 until the broken cochlear endosteum to be a continuous curve again, revealing $n_b = 1.67$. (d) The effect of applying algorithm 5.1 with $n_b = 1.67$ to figure 3.8a, where the distortion of the endosteum beneath the laser ablated crater is corrected.

Having proven the feasibility of the procedure, it is ready to be applied to determine the refractive index of the bony shell of the cochlea, which is a more complicated case. Considering the special geometric shape of the cochlea, it is impossible to separate a large bone sheet from the organ similar as the calibration object from cattle femur shown in figure 5.14. Nevertheless, it is still possible to generate a stair-shaped structure on the cochlea with the CO_2 laser, which can be easily achieved by dividing the planned ablation pattern during the cochleostomy (details refer to section 5.4) into two quasi equal halves and execute one of them first. Acquiring an OCT scan of the channel before proceeding to the second half, the calibration image shown in figure 5.16b can be obtained.

As mentioned at the end of section 5.1.3.1, the discontinuous thickness distribution of overlying bone tissue is the reason for the irregular cochlear endosteum beneath the laser ablated craters in the OCT image such as figure 3.8a. The stair in figure 5.16b is the result of the same phenomenon. Analogous as processing figure 5.15a, algorithm 5.2 was applied to figure 5.16b until the broken cochlear endosteum was connected to be a continuous curve again, as shown in figure 5.16c, revealing $n_b = 1.67$ for porcine cochlea. The distorted OCT scan in figure 3.8a was then used for the examination. As expected, the irregular structures became continuous again after applying the algorithm 5.1 with the obtained refractive index (figure 5.16d).

Discussion For both bovine compact bone tissue and porcine cochlea, the examinations above indicate that the refractive indices determined from the calibration objects are also capable for other specimens of the same kind, even though the specimens are separated from different cattles or pigs. The refractive indices provided by the literatures cited at the beginning of this section also indicate that this optical property does not change significantly between different individuals.

However, slight differences in the range of 0.01-0.02 can be concluded from those researches. Nevertheless, the equation (5.12) guarantees that such a difference will lead to a sub-pixel deviation even in the deepest structure visible in the OCT images. Therefore, the difference between individuals could be neglected in most cases. If in some extreme cases, the difference are not negligible and an anew determination of the refractive index is necessary, the procedure used for processing figure 5.16b can be also applied intra-operatively to determine the refractive index for the particular patient individually.

On the other hand, it can be observed in figure 5.16a that the second boundary between acrylic plate and finger (see figure 5.8f for a global view) shows a stair-shaped distortion under the bone specimen tip. The reason for this distortion is that the refractive index compensation proposed in algorithm 5.1 is only designed for single layer case, which regards all pixels beneath the air-sample surface to be bone tissue, while figure 5.8f consists of multiple layers.

For the case of laser-cochleostomy, the bony shell of the cochlea is the only tissue layer between the air and endosteum, so that algorithm 5.1 is reasonable. For the multilayer situation, if the boundaries between the layers and the refractive indices of each single layer are known, the algorithm 5.1 can also be applied to each single layer by regarding the successive tissue boundaries as the air-sample interface in our case. The determination of multiple layer boundaries and the corresponding refractive indices is however challenging. This topic is not the focus of this thesis and will hence not be discussed in detail.

5.1.4 Conclusion

In this section, the three artefacts observed in the example of figure 5.1, namely stripe noises, fan distortion and uncompensated refractive index of bone tissue, are analysed in detail and corrected accordingly. Workflow for detecting of the most superficial air-sample surface with high efficiency and simple parametrization is also proposed.

A methodology using OCT itself to determine the refractive index of bone tissue with the accuracy of two digits after the decimal point is developed, which does not require any special equipments and expertise in optical engineering. After the elimination of artefacts, especially the geometric distortion correction, the structures in the OCT images are now aligned to the correct position, which is an indispensable precondition for the segmentation of the cochlear endosteum.

Notice that the horizontal stripe noise in figure 5.1 is curved after the subsequent geometric distortion correction (see figure 5.8f and 5.16a) and the horizontal sum and intra-line deviation based noise detection mechanism introduced in section 5.1.1.2 will no more be able to detect the noisy lines in this case. Therefore, the stripe noise suppression should always be applied before the correction of the other two distortions, while the sequence of fan distortion correction and refractive index compensation does not matter.

5.2 Image Quality Enhancement

In the previous section, procedure for determination of the sample surface position was developed. Obviously, if the cochlear endosteum can be further detected in the OCT scans, the thickness profile of the residual bone layer above it can be calculated intuitively. However, although the feasibility studies (refer to section 3.2.1) have proven that the endosteum is visible in OCT images, the structure is unfortunately an edge-weak boundary and its segmentation in the original OCT scans without any preprocess will be difficult.

Instead of trying to detect the structure immediately, efforts were made in order to improve the image quality and enhance the edges, which may reduce the complicity of the critical structure segmentation. The procedure is divided into two steps: light attenuation compensation and speckle noise reduction, which will be handled in the following sections.

5.2.1 Compensation of Light Attenuation

Light Attenuation in OCT Images As introduced in section 3.1.1, OCT works with the pulse-echo mechanism and measures the intensity of echo back reflected from the sample. Due to the scattering in other directions and absorption by the tissue, the fraction of the incident measuring beam that is able to come back to the detector of OCT decreases with the increasing penetration depth into the sample.

This phenomenon leads to the attenuation of the echo intensity along the A-scans beneath the sample surface (example see figure 5.10b). Therefore, the OCT images always show a general tendency that the structures get weaker and weaker in the vertical direction, which is also the main reason for the limited imaging depth of OCT in biological tissues.

Figure 5.17a shows an example OCT image of a formalin fixed bone specimen isolated from human skull. A quasi horizontal membranous structure can be observed beneath the sample surface. Due to the light attenuation in the overlying bone tissue, the structure is rather weak, especially in the left half where the bone is thicker. No doubt, such a phenomenon makes the recognition of the structure of interest more difficult, no matter manually or automatically. A compensation of the light attenuation is therefore crucial for the detection of the endosteum.

Considering the similarity between OCT and ultrasound imaging, Girard et al. [GSEM11] have adopted the method for sound attenuation compensation in ultrasonography proposed by Hughes and Duck [HD97] to compensate the light attenuation in OCT images.

Compensation Method The basic idea of this approach is, instead of directly assigning the intensity $I_{\mathrm{r}}(z)$ of the echo from depth z to the corresponding pixel $\mathrm{px}(z)$ in the observed A-scan, the reflectance $\gamma(z)$ of the substance at depth z is assigned to it, denoting how many percent of the incident light that reaches depth z will be reflected back. $\gamma(z)$ is obviously an inherent property of the material which depends only on the local change of refractive indices according to equation (5.10). The resulting pixel values are hence independent of the back-reflected echo intensity and the attenuation in the image is thus compensated. This procedure will be formally described in the following.

The reflectance is simply defined by the ratio $\gamma(z) = I_{\mathrm{r}}(z)/I_{\mathrm{i}}(z)$, where $I_{\mathrm{i}}(z)$ denotes the total intensity of the incident light that has reached depth z and can be estimated by the integral

$$I_{\mathrm{i}}(z) = 2\int_{z}^{\infty} I(u)\mathrm{d}u$$

Consequently, the new value of the pixel $\mathrm{px}(z)$ can be written as

$$\mathrm{px}(z) = \gamma(z) = \frac{I_{\mathrm{r}}(z)}{2\displaystyle\int_{z}^{\infty} I_{\mathrm{r}}(u)\mathrm{d}u} \tag{5.13}$$

Moreover, in order to enhance the contrast of the pixels, Girard et al. have further squared the intensity terms in equation (5.13), yielding

$$\mathrm{px}(z) = \frac{I_{\mathrm{r}}^{2}(z)}{2\displaystyle\int_{z}^{\infty} I_{\mathrm{r}}^{2}(u)\mathrm{d}u} \tag{5.14}$$

In order to apply equation (5.14) to an $m \times n$ image, it is further rewritten in the discrete form

$$\mathrm{px}(i,j) = \frac{I_{\mathrm{r}}^{2}(i,j)}{2\displaystyle\sum_{k=i}^{m} I_{\mathrm{r}}^{2}(k,j)} \tag{5.15}$$

where $1 \leq i \leq m$ and $1 \leq j \leq n$ and $I_{\mathrm{r}}(i,j)$ denotes the echo intensity in the uncompensated OCT image. Figure 5.17b shows the effect of applying equation (5.15) to figure 5.17a. Compared to the original image, the brightness of the pixels are more uniform beneath the bone surface in the compensated one and the image quality is significantly improved, where the membranous structures are much clearer and easier to be recognized.

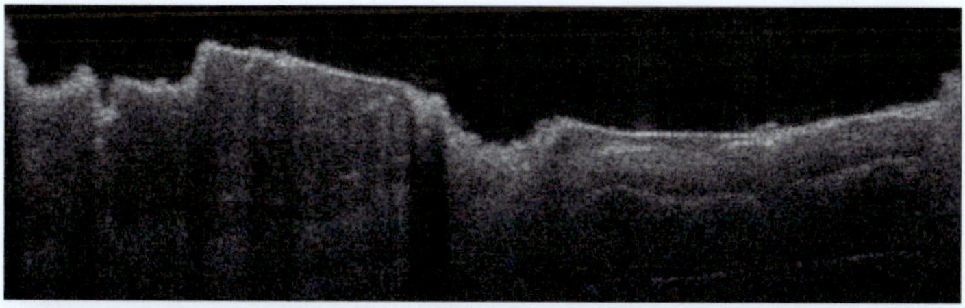

(a)

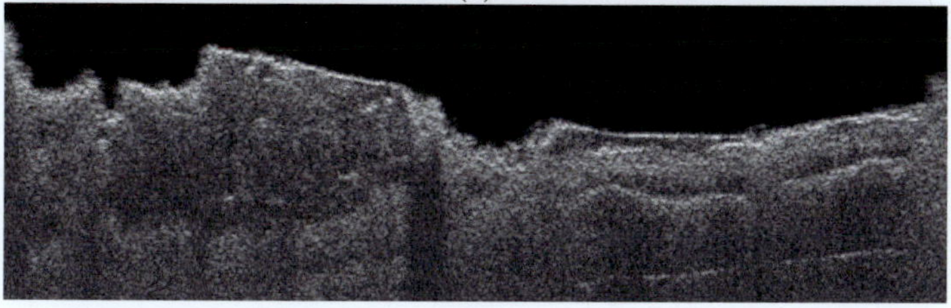

(b)

Figure 5.17: OCT scan of a formalin fixed human skull bone specimen (a) before and (b) after the compensation of light attenuation.

Boundary Emphasising Effect Reviewing the analysis of equation (5.10) in section 5.1.3.3, it can be concluded that the more drastic is the local change in the refractive indices $\eta(z)$, the larger will the reflectance $\gamma(z)$ be, corresponding to brighter pixels $\mathrm{px}(i, j)$ after the light attenuation compensation defined by equations (5.13)-(5.15). Moreover, η are often very different in the media intersecting the tissue boundaries, for example at the most superficial air-bone interface and the critical bone-endosteum-perilymph boundary, resulting in larger $\mathrm{px}(i, j)$ accordingly. On the contrary, the difference of η inside the bone layer, air, and perilymph is less significant, which are hence corresponding to smaller $\mathrm{px}(i, j)$. As a result, the relevant boundaries are expected to be emphasised after the application of equation (5.15).

An example is shown in figure 5.18, where two chambers (scalae) can be observed in the OCT images. It can be immediately discovered that after applying the light attenuation compensation, the bone-endosteum-perilymph interfaces in both Scalae remain bright structures while the brightness in the overlying bone layer and underlying perilymph is reduced. As a result, the contrast of the critical structures are significantly enhanced in the post-compensation image, which will be advantageous to the automatic boundary detection.

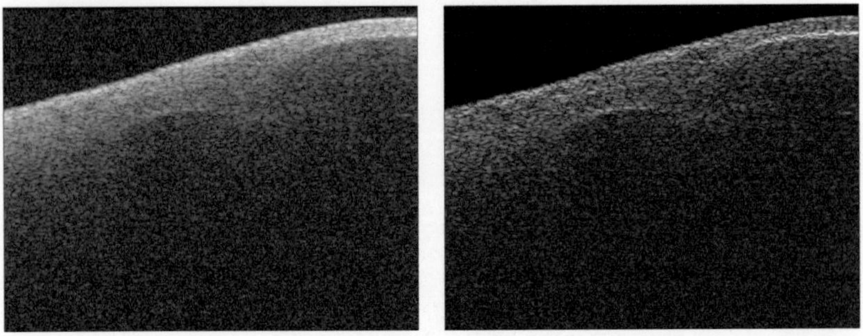

(a) (b)

Figure 5.18: Boundary emphasising effect of equation (5.15): (a) original OCT scan of a fresh porcine cochlea and (b) the light attenuation compensated scan after applying equation (5.15).

5.2.2 Speckle Noise Reduction

In addition to the light attenuation, another major weakness of OCT is the so called *speckle noise*, which is an inherited phenomenon from the laser technology, known as *laser speckle*. This phenomenon was discovered shortly after the invention of laser during the 1960's, where dark and bright spots are formed by the laser beam reflected back from a rough surface with a distinctive granular or mottled appearance [AJ63]. These spots have no obvious relationship to the texture of the surface and change their patten whenever the surface is slightly moved [RG97].

The speckles are caused by random interference between reflected waves that are mutually coherent, which is also a fundamental property of signals and images acquired by all types of narrowband detection systems including radar, ultrasound and radio astronomy [SXY99]. On the other hand, as its name suggests, the interferometry based optical *coherence* tomography relies on the spatial and temporal coherence of the echo back-reflected from the target tissue. Therefore, the speckles are inherent to OCT images, carrying information about the micro-structures beneath the tissue surface meanwhile also acting as a source of noise.

Taking the OCT images in figure 5.18 as example and magnifying the bone-endosteum-perilymph interfaces of both chambers, as shown in figure 5.19, irregular textures consist of bright spots separated by narrow cracks and dark spots arise overall beneath the bone surface.

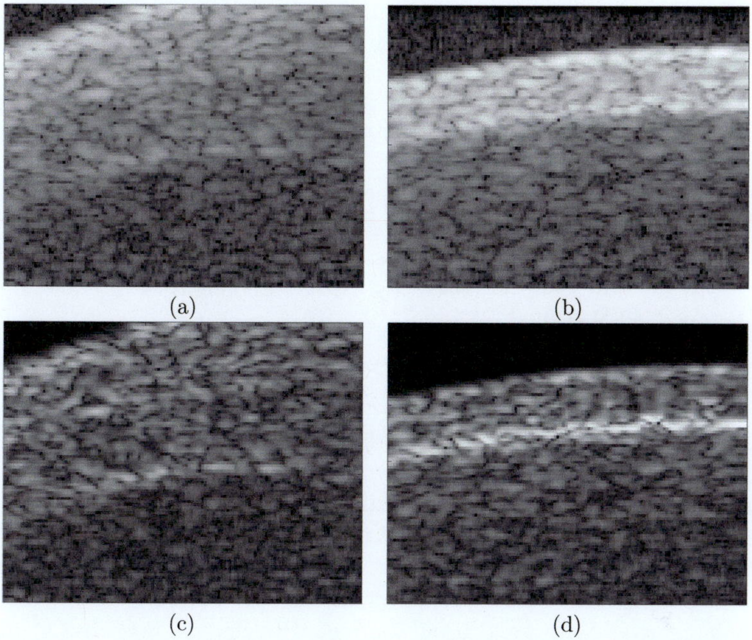

Figure 5.19: Magnified view of the bone-endosteum-perilymph interfaces of both chambers in figure 5.18, which suffer from speckle noises: (a-b) left and right chambers in the original scan; (c-d) left and right chambers in the post-compensation scan, where speckle noises are also emphasised.

These textures are exactly the so-called speckles. Despite the high resolution of the OCT, speckle noises compromise the ability to resolve the relevant boundaries. For instance, in figure 5.19a-b, speckles crossing over the tissue interfaces have blurred the boundaries at multiple positions, hindering a unique boundary detection, especially at the left chamber (figure 5.19a) where the boundary is less significant due to thicker overlying bone tissue and stronger light attenuation. As a result, even a manual segmentation of the critical structure is difficult.

Although the light attenuation compensation method proposed by Girard et al. has improved the macroscopic contrast of the critical structures in figure 5.18b, its boundary emphasising effect leads to a side effect that the contrast of the speckles are also increased after applying equation (5.15), as shown in figure 5.19c-d. High gray value gradients will occur along the contours of the speckles, which have negative influence on any segmentation techniques that take gradients into account and counteract the image quality enhancement brought by the method. A speckle noise reduction method is therefore necessary.

5.2.2.1 Speckle Noise Reduction Techniques: An Overview

Speckle noise reduction has been since years an important research topic in the context of OCT. According to the working principles, major speckle noise reduction approaches nowadays can be categorized into two groups: single-frame based algorithms and multi-frame averaging techniques [FLN+12].

Single-Frame Based Algorithms The methods of the first group try to adopt mature algorithmic denoising techniques in the field of digital image processing to OCT scans directly. Typical approaches of this category rely on analysing local image properties and corresponding post-processing, for example the wavelet based filtering [CYV00, AKF04, OBD+07, CFF09], general Bayesian least squares estimation [WMBC10], anisotropic diffusion algorithms [YA02, PB09] etc. Dozens of related researches have been conducted in diverse branches of digital image processing and can be used for reference while designing the algorithm for OCT images.

The main shortcoming of these approaches is that they were originally designed for general digital image processing, which do not take the special properties of OCT into account. As stated above, the speckles in OCT images are information carrying and source of noise simultaneously. The power spectral densities of the signal-carrying and signal-degrading speckles are hence overlapped [SXY99], which are difficult to be distinguished by analysis in spatial domain directly. Through the filtering and estimation in the local neighbourhood, some loss of useful information is inevitable after applying theses methods. A trade-off between speckle reduction and spatial resolution has to be made [KHCS10].

Another drawback is, all these algorithms focus on processing two-dimensional images, where most approaches are already quite complicated in this case and consume several seconds to minutes for processing a single OCT image on state of the art computer platforms [WMBC10, FLN+12] [5]. For the three-dimensional case, the approaches have to be iteratively applied to several hundred frames in the 3D volume, which will lead to unacceptable computing time and further adaptation and optimization for the 3D case are necessary.

Multi-Frame Averaging Techniques Compared to the single-frame based approaches, the multi-frame averaging techniques work in a quite different way, also known as *compounding*. As mentioned, a slight movement between the laser and target surface can already result in different laser speckle patterns which are less correlated. By simple arithmetic averaging of these decorrelated patterns, the level of coherence in the OCT scan can be reduced accordingly and the speckles are hence suppressed. Taking advantage of such an effect, the main idea of compounding techniques is to average multiple scans of the same object acquired under varying conditions. The techniques of these group are much efficient than those of the first group and suitable for processing both two- and three-dimensional scans spontaneously.

Despite the simplicity and efficiency of the calculation, generation of decorrelated OCT scans is however challenging. A common approach is the spatial compounding by acquiring multiple OCT scans of the same object from different incident angles [Sch97, BR00, IBT03, DVO+07, WR09]; another possibility is to utilize measuring beam within different light frequency bands, yielding the frequency compounding technique [SXY99, PGL+03]. However, both spatial and frequency compounding techniques require significant modification to the optical components of OCT system, so that expertise in optical engineering is essential. Furthermore, the modification of the optics in both cases is accompanied with loss of axial resolution [SXY99] from the optics side, which severely limits the application of these techniques in practice.

Kennedy et al. [KHCS10, KCH+11] have hence proposed another compounding approach, namely strain compounding, providing a different thread of generating the uncorrelated speckles. Instead of modifying the optical components, the authors have tried to compress the sample with

[5] A comparison between performance of diverse algorithms can be found in [WMBC10].

different strain, resulting in changing optical properties of the target tissue and changing speckle patterns accordingly. Without modification of the optics, the original axial resolution of the utilized OCT system will be retained in each acquired scan. By proper alignment and averaging of the obtained speckle patterns, incoherent OCT scans can be obtained without loss in spatial resolution.

The disadvantage of the compounding techniques is also obvious, which requires multiple scans of the same object. Although the averaging itself is simple, the acquisition of the multiple scans is however time consuming. Furthermore, special modification of the OCT system or sample is necessary in order to generate decorrelated scans, which are not always possible in many situations, for example the strain compounding is not able to be applied on rigid bony cochlea in our case.

5.2.2.2 History Compounding

Analysis Although not capable of acquiring OCT images on bony tissue, the strain compounding reveals that if uncorrelated scans could be generated without modifying the optics, compounding techniques can achieve speckle noise reduction without loss in spatial resolution. Contrarily, a trade-off between speckle reduction effect and spatial resolution is inherent to single frame based algorithms.

On the other hand, as conceived in figure 3.10, during the process of OCT guided laser-cochleostomy, the laser ablation and OCT scanning have to be executed in turn, so that several tens of 3D OCT volume will be acquired and processed online. Therefore, the efficiency of the speckle noise reduction method is another key issue.

Taking no account of the time overhead for data acquisition, the arithmetic averaging of the acquired OCT volume is significantly more efficient than the complicated algorithms of the single frame based approaches. Consequently, a compounding based technique is more promising for the control loop to be developed. However, none of the existing compounding techniques can be applied for our case directly and an adaptation of them or even a completely new technique is expected.

A trivial idea is therefore to adapt the conventional spatial compounding techniques. Traditionally, the incident angles were altered by specially designed optics, which however sacrifice the spatial resolution of the

OCT. Alternatively, a robot assisted OCT scanning system similar to the robot assisted laser osteotomy (refer to section 2.3.1) can be easily realized by coupling the OCT to a robot, so that the direction of the incident measuring beam can be readily changed by relocating the OCT optics with the robot, as illustrated in figure 5.20a. Thus, the modification in the optical parts of the OCT system is no more necessary and its high spatial resolution will hence be retained.

However, supposing the spatial compounding requires N extra scans acquired from different directions for generating a speckle noise suppressed scan, the total number of the OCT scans required during the whole ablation process will be tremendously increased for N times accordingly, which makes the efficiency issue more critical. Moreover, with the increasing channel depth, the tilted optical path from the OCT to the channel bottom will be blocked by the channel lip. The imaging of the micro-structures beneath the channel bottom will be more difficult in such a case. Consequently, the robot assisted spatial compounding is not a suitable solution for the desired control loop and a new concept of compounding technique is necessary.

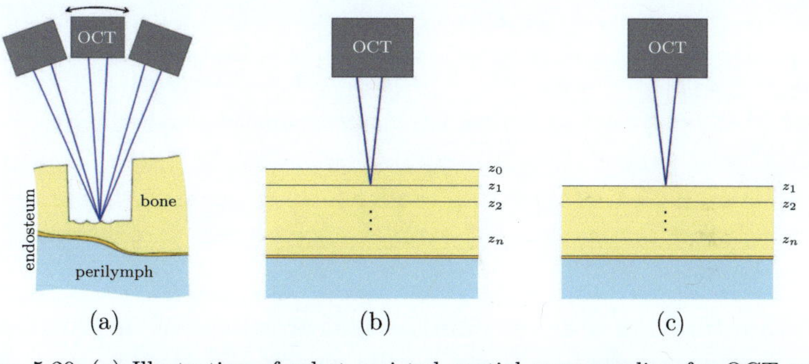

Figure 5.20: (a) Illustration of robot assisted spatial compounding for OCT scan, where the incident angle of the measuring beam is changed by relocating the OCT with the help of a robot. (b-c) Illustration of the reducing bone thickness over the structure of interest during the process of cochleostomy, which will result in varying speckle patterns in the acquired OCT scans.

The existing compounding techniques reveal that the key point of such approaches is to generate uncorrelated speckle patterns of the same object, which can be achieved by changing the conditions during the OCT scan acquisition, including incident angles, light frequency bands and even compression of the sample. Hence, how to make reasonable alternations to the acquisition conditions is the main consideration while designing a new compounding technique.

Notice that the thickness of the bone tissue above the cochlear endosteum or other structures of interest is reducing with the increasing channel depth of the cochleostomy. Divide the overlying bone tissue virtually into thin layers, as illustrated in figure 5.20b-c. The layer z_0z_1 in sub-figure b is ablated in sub-figure c. Obviously, the measuring beam from the OCT has to penetrate the layer z_0z_1 before reaching the depth z_1 in sub-figure b. For the situation in sub-figure c, the original measuring beam can arrive z_1 directly without passing through any other structures. Due to the scattering, reflection and absorption inside the layer z_0z_1, the wavefront of the measuring beam reaching the depth z_1 will be definitively different in both cases. In other words, the measuring beams reaching z_1 are not the same one in sub-figure b and c. Actually, not only at the depth z_1 but also any $z \geq z_1$, the measuring beams are different in the two situations.

On the other hand, the speckles are the result of the spatial and temporal coherence of the back reflected measuring beam. With the changing measuring beam, varying speckle patterns of the same structure are expected, yielding the proposition 5.4. By simple averaging of these patterns, a novel compounding concept can be conceived and the speckle noise of the observed structure could be suppressed accordingly.

Proposition 5.4. *The speckle patterns of a same structure will be changed when the thickness of overlying bone tissue is reduced.*

Observation In order to examine the correctness of the proposition 5.4, feasibility experiment was conducted on a bovine compact bone sheet with manually polished flat surface and a thickness of circa 1 mm. Two questions have to be answered by this experiment:

i. Do the speckle patterns change as expected while the thickness of overlying bone tissue is reduced?

ii. How much should the channel be deepened between the acquisition of two successive scans in order to generate significantly different speckle patterns?

A dummy channel was drilled on the bone sheet manually with a diamond burr (diameter 1.2 mm) under the OCT scanner directly and

OCT scans were acquired at different channel depths. The specimen was clamped to an aluminium slab underneath in order to keep it fixed during the drilling process and the bone-aluminium interface was regarded as a dummy critical structure.

It was discovered that a channel depth increase of only 15-20 μm can already lead to a remarkable change in the speckle patterns as expected, for example the selected region beneath the drilled channel in figure 5.21a-b [6]. Contrarily, the speckle patterns outside the drilled channel remain identical in both scans. It can hence be concluded that the ablation of the overlaying bone tissue is the only reason for the change in the speckle patterns.

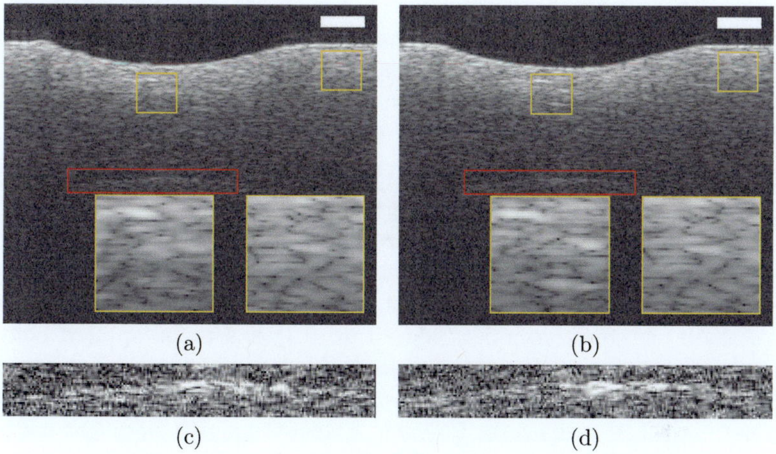

Figure 5.21: (a-b) Two successive scans of the channel bottom during the drilling experiment on a bovine compact bone specimen, where the channel in (b) is 15-20 μm (roughly 2-3 pixels) deeper than in (a). The speckle patterns in the same region beneath the channel (see the yellow regions on the left in both images and the corresponding zoomed views below) are remarkably changed but remain identical in the region outside the channel (the right ones), white bars=200 μm in air. (c-d) Magnified view of the red regions near the bone-aluminium interface in (a-b), where a significant change in speckle patterns can be observed. White balance in (c-d) has been adjusted for better printing effect.

[6] The example images are original scans without any post-processing, so that the refractive index of bone tissue is uncompensated, leading to an axial shift of the speckles for 1-3 pixels. Nevertheless, such an artefact has very little influence on the shape of the speckles and does not hinder the investigation of the speckle patterns.

Further observation of the dummy critical structure was made, where the regions near the bone-aluminium interface are magnified and shown in sub-figure c-d. Although the speckles at this depth are less clear due to the relatively thicker overlying bone layer (circa 700-800 μm), the difference in speckle patterns are still clearly visible. This phenomenon indicates that a slight change of the most superficial bone layer can already affect the speckle patterns of the structures deeply located beneath the tissue surface. The proposition 5.4 is therefore correct.

Concept The proposition 5.4 and example shown in figure 5.21 reveal that uncorrelated speckle patterns of any structures beneath the bone surface can be simply generated during the process of cochleostomy with the increasing channel depth. Taking advantage of this phenomenon, an intuitive compounding technique has been be developed based on averaging of the OCT scans recording the history of the channel ablation process, namely *history compounding.*

According to equation (5.8), the varying overlying bone thickness d will lead to changing distortion Δl due to uncompensated refractive index, resulting in misalignment of the structures in different historical scans. For example, the straight bone-aluminium boundaries are shown curved in figure 5.21 due to the shape of the channel bottom. Therefore, compensation of refractive index (algorithm 5.1) has to be applied before the averaging so that the speckles from the same structures in different historical scans are aligned together. Contrarily, the fan distortion (refer to section 5.1.2) is constant for each A-scan. Hence, it does not matter whether this artefact is corrected before or after the compounding.

Figure 5.22 illustrates the concept of history compounding, where the flat bone-aluminium interfaces are straight lines again and aligned to the same position in every historical scan after the refractive index compensation. Reviewing the OCT A-scan reconstruction introduced in section 3.1.5, the pixel values are only additive after the logarithm. Meanwhile, the dynamic range adjustment by clipping makes the scalar of the gray values to be non-linear. Therefore, the averaging must be performed between these two steps.

In order to ensure storage efficiency, the resulting scans will not be stored in memory directly but immediately added to a volume buffer storing the sum of all preceding scans. The OCT volume with suppressed speckle noises can be intuitively obtained by averaging this sum.

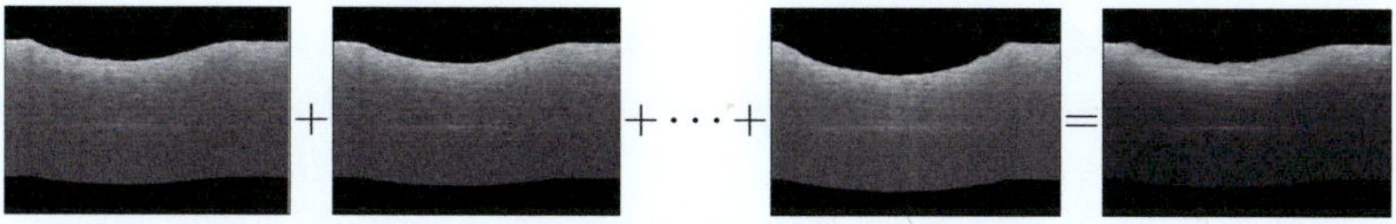

Figure 5.22: Concept of history compounding: align the speckles by applying refractive index compensation (algorithm 5.1) to each historical scan and calculate their arithmetic average.

Evaluation The effect of history compounding is demonstrated in figure 5.23. Compared with the original scan, the speckle noises beneath the drilled channel are significantly reduced in sub-figure b. The bone-aluminium interface which is regarded as a dummy critical structure appears to be a sharper continuous line in the post-compounding scan while some segments of the boundary are fairly blurred by speckles noises in sub-figure a. Similar to figure 5.21a-b, the speckle patterns outside the drilled channel remain almost unchanged after the history compounding[7], indicating the image quality enhancement lies only in the changing overlying bone layers.

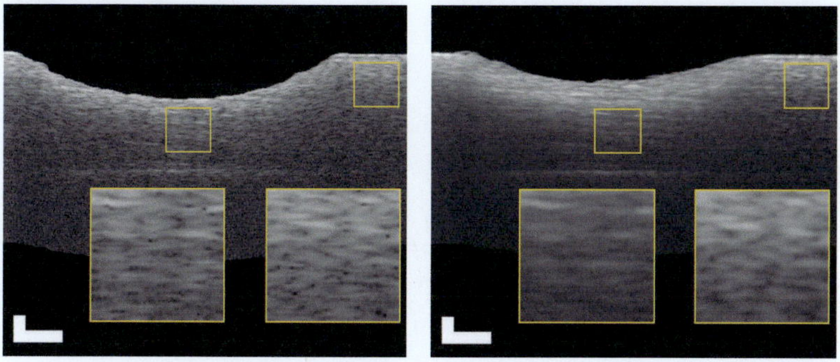

(a) (b)

Figure 5.23: Effect of history compounding: (a) original scan after refractive index compensation and (b) after history compounding with six previous historical scans, where the speckle noises in the regions beneath the channel (left) and near the bone-aluminium interface are significantly reduced, meanwhile remain almost unchanged outside the channel (right), bars=200 μm.

[7] The speckles in the selected region seem to be a little blurred in the post-compounding scan. The reason is that a movement of the bone specimen on micrometer scale cannot be avoided during the drilling process with a diamond burr despite of the fixation, which results in slight shift of the speckles and blur the averaged image.

Further experiments were conducted on fresh porcine cochlea in order to examine the effectiveness of history compounding for the real application on cochlear endosteum, where the cochleostomy was also performed manually with a 1.2 mm diamond burr. The original scan after refractive index compensation is shown in figure 5.24a. Similar as the previous example, the speckle noises are significantly suppressed after applying history compounding (sub-figure b). Moreover, by averaging the historical scans, the approach is no more limited by a single scan but compounds information about the critical structures from diverse historical scans. In this particular example, the right part of the endosteum, which can be barely seen in the original scan, is supplemented by the compounding and becomes very clear in the resulting image. Any single frame based approach is not able to achieve such an enhancement.

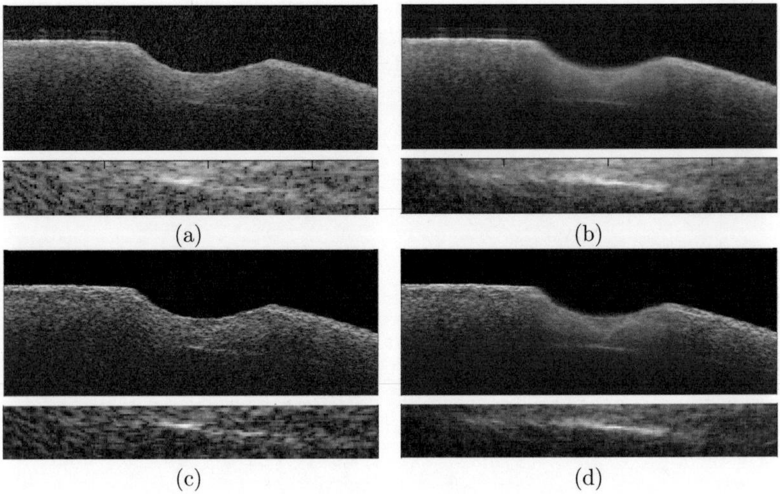

Figure 5.24: Effect of combining history compounding (HC) and light attenuation compensation (LAC) on an OCT scan of a fresh porcine cochlea: (a) the original scan; (b) after HC; (c) after LAC; (d) after applying HC first and then LAC. The magnified regions of interest near the cochlear endosteum are shown below each image.

It is further noticed that the contrast of the transition from bone to endosteum is lower than that from endosteum to perilymph in sub-figure b. Taking advantage of the boundary emphasising effect, the light attenuation compensation (section 5.2.1) might be a solution to improve the contrast. It is therefore applied to the compounded image as well as the original one for comparison, as shown in figure 5.24c-d. As expected, although the compensation alone can improve the contrast of the structures, it can however only emphasis the structures that are already visible to some extent in the original image. The right part of the endosteum is still not clear in the compensated image (sub-figure c). Nevertheless, after applying this method to the compounded scan in sub-figure b, the contrast of the endosteum is considerably enhanced (sub-figure d). Compared with the original scan shown in sub-figure a, the edge-weak cochlear endosteum becomes now an edge-strong boundary and can be uniquely recognized, indicating the feasibility of the combination of these two techniques.

To give an quantitative evaluation of the image quality enhancement in the above examples, the contrast to noise ratio (CNR) and signal to noise ratio (SNR) within the regions of interest near the bone-aluminium boundary (figure 5.23) and cochlear endosteum (figure 5.24) are calculated according to the following equations [WMBC10, FLN+12]:

$$\mathrm{CNR} = \frac{|\mu_{\mathrm{f}} - \mu_{\mathrm{b}}|}{\sqrt{\sigma_{\mathrm{f}}^2 + \sigma_{\mathrm{b}}^2}} \qquad \mathrm{SNR} = \frac{\mu_{\mathrm{f}}}{\sigma_{\mathrm{b}}}$$

where μ and σ indicate the mean values and standard deviation of the pixels in the chosen regions. The subscripts f and b denote the foreground and background respectively. The results are listed in table 5.1.

Table 5.1: Quantitative evaluation of image quality enhancement after applying history compounding (HC), light attenuation compensation (LAC) and HC+LAC (Mixed) to the examples in figures 5.23a and 5.24a.

image	criterion	original	HC	LAC	Mixed
figure 5.23a	CNR	0.61	1.32	0.92	1.46
	SNR	4.06	9.38	6.48	15.01
figure 5.24a	CNR	1.17	1.98	1.35	2.21
	SNR	4.16	10.87	4.84	12.74

From which can be concluded that both history compounding and light attenuation compensation can enhance the CNR and SNR in the regions of interest. Similar as the above subjective judgement, the history compounding shows a better performance than light attenuation compensation while applying the two techniques separately. The combination of both techniques provides a significant improvement in both criteria.

Discussion The experiments above demonstrate that history compounding combined with the light attenuation compensation is a very effective speckle noise reduction technique to improve the image quality of the cochlear endosteum. Compared to the other speckle noise reduction techniques introduced in section 5.2.2.1, the new approach has the following advantages:

i. No trade-off between spatial resolution and speckle noise reduction effect needed.
ii. Takes full advantage of the historical scans acquired during the process of laser-cochleostomy and requires no extra image acquisition overhead.
iii. Extremely simple calculation and requires almost no extra computational cost.
iv. Intuitive deployment without any hardware modification.

Considering the working principle, history compounding is also capable of monitoring other kind of hard tissue ablation with almost any kind of OCT systems. However, this also brings the main limitation of the approach that it works only for the situation with a changing tissue layer. It is therefore excluded for routine clinical inspection without tissue ablation.

As mentioned, compounding techniques require aligning the speckles from the same structure together. In the above examples, all samples were fixed and static to the OCT system. A dynamic case with relative movement between the target area and the OCT scanning optics will be handled in section 6.2.

5.3 Segmentation of Cochlear Endosteum

After the image quality enhancement of the OCT scans, the cochlear endosteum becomes now an edge-strong structure in the images. The succeeding segmentation is therefore much easier. Obviously, only the endosteum position beneath the bottom of the insertion channel plays a role to the subsequent ablation. Therefore, a three-dimensional cuboid volume of interest is defined centred at the axis of the insertion channel and covers the whole channel. Figure 5.25a shows a frame within the chosen volume of interest as example.

Analysis Observing the structure to be segmented in figure 5.25a, it can be discovered that the endosteum is an edge-strong boundary showing a dark-bright-dark appearance in the enhanced image. Therefore, the voxels on the visible part of the endosteum can be easily detected by calculating the gray value gradients.

Due to the limited imaging depth of OCT into bone tissue, the structure gets weaker where the overlying bone tissue becomes thicker, so that the extracted voxels on the visible part of the endosteum do not form a boundary crossing over the whole volume of interest and hence do not divide the frame into separated parts either. Therefore, among the diverse techniques introduced in section 4.2, the region based approaches and morphological watersheds segmentation are excluded from the candidates list.

Moreover, with the varying thickness of the overlying bone tissue within the volume of interest, the length of the visible part of the endosteum is also changing from frame to frame. The graph based edge linking approach and parametric deformable models will only be able to precisely detect the visible part of the endosteum while the extracted surface outside the visible part will probably be drawn to wrong positions by other stronger structure inside the bone layer. Therefore, neither of these two techniques are capable for the detection.

For such a case where the structure to be detected is only partially visible, an A prior model based segmentation is vital, which can predict the invisible parts by the model. A typical approach of this kind is the active shape model. However, considering the diameter of cochlea on centimetre scale and the channel diameter of only circa 1 mm, the volume of interest is actually a small part on the bony shell of the scala tympani, as marked in figure 5.25b. Therefore, the visible voxels on the endosteum actually cover only a very small part of the curved surface, providing no significant feature points. As a result, it will be difficult to establish an appropriate training set for the model, which prevents deploying the method for our case.

The remaining feasible candidate technique is hence the edge linking using parametric surface. Considering that the cochlea endosteum is locally a regular curved surface crossing over the whole volume of interest marked in figure 5.25b, an intuitive idea is to describe the structure using bi-cubic B-spline surface (refer to [PBP02]) due to its simple calculation and high flexibility. Meanwhile, the B-splines also ensure a minimal strain energy along the extracted surface with a C^2 continuity.

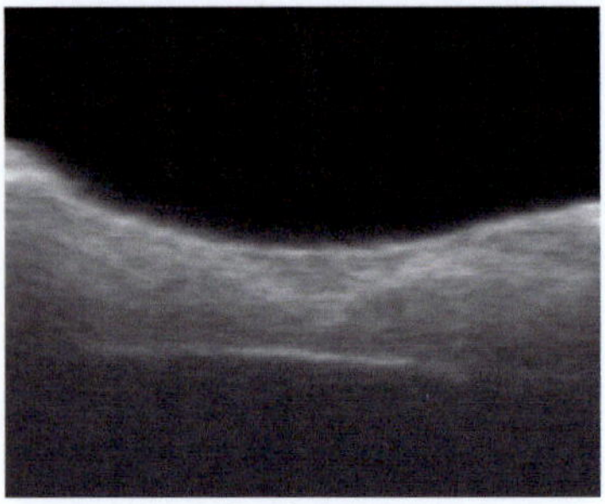

(a)

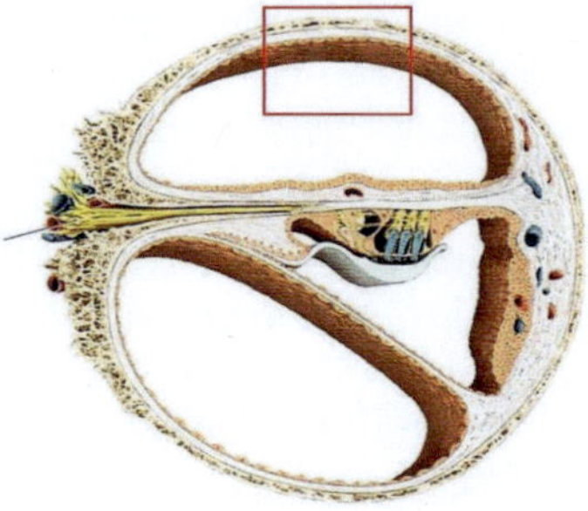

(b)

Figure 5.25: (a) An example of a frame in the volume of interest with cochlear endosteum partially visible. (b) Illustration of the chosen volume of interest on the cochlea (marked with red box), original inscribed image see figure 2.1b.

Workflow As analysed above, the first step is to calculate the gradient in the image. Particularly, if the angle between the optical axis of OCT and the surface normal of the cochlear endosteum is too large, most measuring beam is not able to be reflected back to the OCT detector and makes it impossible to imaging the structure. Hence, the OCT is always oriented so, that the incident angle is not very large with respect to the normal of the endosteum. Moreover, due to the scanning mechanism of OCT (see figure 3.2), the lateral and axial resolution of OCT scans are independent to each other. By increasing the scanning density (number of A-scans per millimetre), any inclined structures can be dilated in the horizontal direction, reducing its slope in the OCT scan. Consequently, it is ensured that the principle direction of the endosteum is horizontal and it is enough to observe only the vertical gradient of the image.

The routine procedure is to apply the vertical Sobel operator (equation (4.4) left) to the given frame. In addition, the operator is extended to the third dimension and the gradient of the current frame is a weighted sum of three neighbouring frames. The centre frame is given a weight of 2 and the two neighbours are given a weight of 1. Figure 5.26a shows the vertical gradient map of the input volume of interest (figure 5.25a). Furthermore, it is ensured that the bone surface is not tangent to the endosteum and there exists some non-zero vertical distance between them. Therefore, the gradients near the surface are forced to zero.

The endosteum has a dark-bright-dark appearance in the enhanced OCT image from top to bottom. Therefore, the gradient map always has negative-zero-positive values near the boundary, corresponding to the black-gray-white structure in figure 5.26a. To emphasis this structure, the mask below is applied to the image using linear spatial filtering (equation (4.2)). The weight denote that the bright to dark boundary beneath the endosteum is stronger than the dark to bright one above.

$$\begin{pmatrix} -1 & -1 & -1 & -1 & -1 \\ -1 & -1 & -1 & -1 & -1 \\ 0 & 0 & 0 & 0 & 0 \\ 2 & 2 & 2 & 2 & 2 \\ 2 & 2 & 2 & 2 & 2 \end{pmatrix} \tag{5.16}$$

The result of the filtering is shown in sub-figure b, where the endosteum is clearly emphasised. A global thresholding in the whole volume of interest is then applied to generate a binary volume, where the threshold is automatically determined by the same histogram analysis method introduced in figure 5.4b. As stated in remark 5.1, the A-scans polluted by specular highlights contain no more usable information about the internal structures of the sample. Therefore, all voxels from the columns marked as invalid are eliminated before proceeding to the next step.

The result of the filtering also have large values at non-endosteum structures in sub-figure b, some are even almost as bright as the weaker left part of the endosteum. Such voxels will also pass the thresholding. Nevertheless, the endosteum is the dominating structure and a connectivity test is performed to the binary volume. Only the voxels in the largest connected component are regarded as valid candidates, as shown in sub-figure c. A weighted bi-cubic B-spline surface fitting of the candidate point cloud is then calculated, where the values of the candidate voxels after the filtering using equation (5.16) are regarded as their weights. The obtained surface $z = M(x, y)$ is also plotted in sub-figure c, giving an initial estimation of the critical structure.

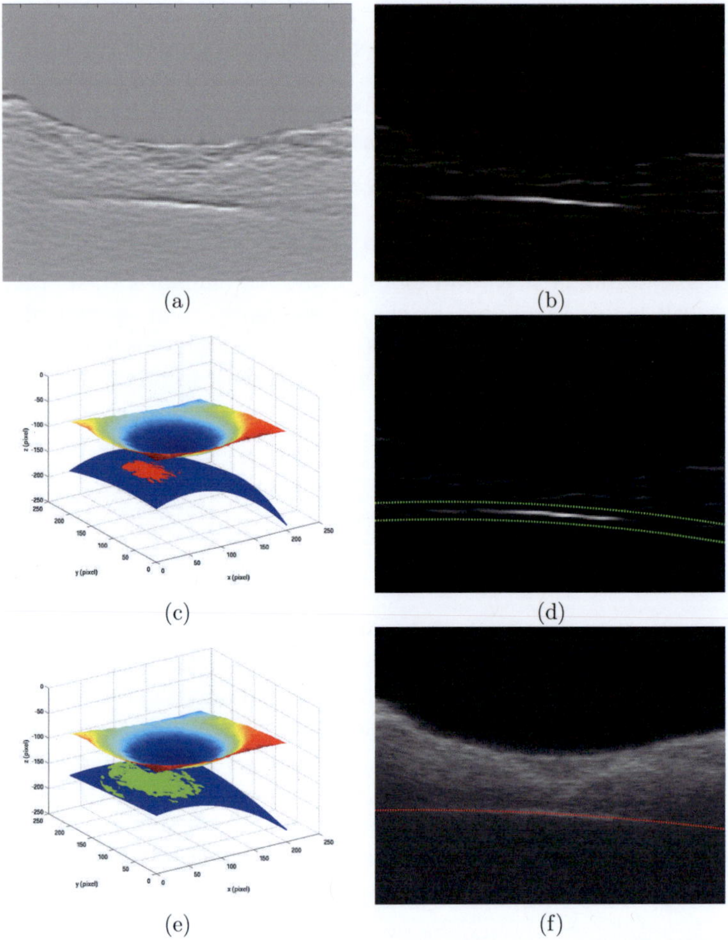

Figure 5.26: Workflow of cochlear endosteum detection using figure 5.25a as example: (a) after applying vertical 3D Sobel operator; (b) after linear spatial filtering using equation (5.16); (c) candidate voxels (red point cloud) after global thresholding and connectivity test. The blue surface is the result of weighted bi-cubic B-spline fitting; (d) the tolerance range (green); (e) candidate voxels (green point cloud) after a second thresholding within the tolerance range and the anew calculated B-spline surface describing the endosteum (blue surface); (f) detected endosteum position in the given frame.

Although the surface $M(x, y)$ fits the candidate voxels very well, it should be noticed that many visible voxels on the endosteum are neglected by the connectivity test and excluded for the fitting. An example is the left part of the endosteum in sub-figure b, which is separated from the strong main part on the right by a weak gap. If such voxels could also be taken into account, a more precise result of the detection is expected. On the other hand, the current B-spline surface is determined based on the strongest voxels on the endosteum. It gives hence a prediction of the endosteum position with certain accuracy within some neighbourhood of the candidate voxels. In other words, the deviation of $M(x, y)$ from the correct position is small if (x, y) is not far from the candidate point cloud.

Based on this consideration, a tolerance range with the thickness of four times of the endosteum thickness is defined above and below the surface, as illustrated in sub-figure d. An anew thresholding is performed within the tolerance range. Thus, more voxels lying on the critical structure that were however excluded for the first round of fitting (for example the left part of the endosteum mentioned above) are now also included, as plotted in sub-figure e. Repeating the weighted bi-cubic B-spline surface fitting, the position and shape of the cochlear endosteum can be finally determined. The sub-figure f shows the final result of the cochlear endosteum detection in the given frame, which precisely matches the visible part of the critical structure, meanwhile gives a prediction of the endosteum position towards both sides for the invisible part. Thus, a three-dimensional model of the critical structure can be established, as shown in figure 5.27.

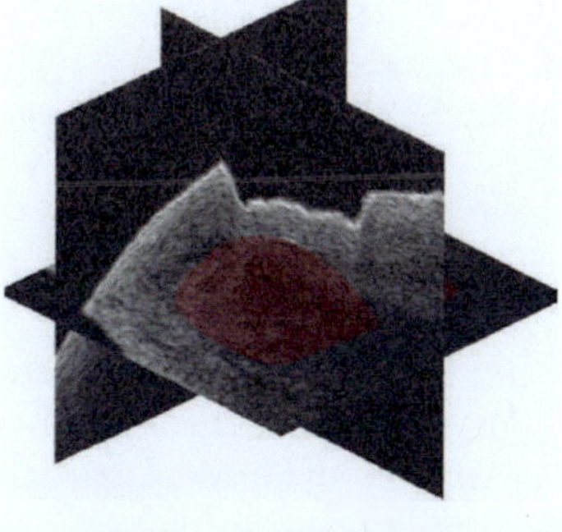

Figure 5.27: The three dimensional model of the endosteal layer (red) reconstructed from the OCT volume.

Discussion The mechanism of the B-spline fitting ensures that the resulting surface is always the optimal bi-cubic surface with minimal square error passing through the given point cloud. The correctness of the endosteum position at its visible part is therefore guaranteed. The fitting also automatically fills the gap between the unconnected visible parts of the endosteum.

However, the accuracy of the position prediction for non-visible part of the endosteum outside the point cloud might decrease with increasing distance to the cloud. Nevertheless, the invisible endosteum also indicates a thick overlying bone tissue and the inaccurate prediction at these positions is temporarily not critical. With the increasing channel depth, more and more parts of the endosteum will become visible, providing more candidate voxels for the fitting. Therefore, an anew segmentation in will improve the accuracy of the prediction for the still invisible part of the critical structure.

5.4 Ablation Planning

Knowing the position of the bone surface and the cochlear endosteum in the OCT scans, a three-dimensional thickness profile of the residual bone tissue above the critical structure can be spontaneously calculated. Based on the bone thickness distribution within the volume of interest, the laser ablation can be planned, where two important parameters have to be determined: the pulse position and pulse duration.

For a formal description, the process of the whole laser-cochleostomy is divided into layers. Each layer contains an *ablation pattern*, which is defined as a set of three-tuples $AP = \{(x_i, y_i; \tau_i)\}$, where (x_i, y_i) and τ_i are the position and pulse duration of the i-th pulse in the current layer.

5.4.1 Ablation Depth-based Strategy

As introduced in section 2.3.1, Kahrs et al. [Kah09] have developed a control mechanism for laser-cochleostomy using conventional video camera. In order to create the cylindrical insertion channel, a virtual ablation depth-based strategy was developed. Before developing our own ablation planning module, this strategy will be analysed first.

Accumulative Depth Without knowing the residual bone thickness distribution, the strategy of Kahrs relies on the channel depth profile within the volume of interest instead, say $D_{M\times N}$. Supposing the laser beam radius is r, for any given point (x_0, y_0) within the insertion channel, the *accumulative depth* of this point is defined as

$$AD(x_0, y_0) = \sum_{|(x,y)-(x_0,y_0)|<r} D(x, y) \tag{5.17}$$

where $|\cdot|$ denotes the distance between the two points. Furthermore, a critical point set P is given, which contains the detected positions where the cochlear endosteum is already exposed to air or perforated, as illustrated in figure 5.28a. No more pulses are allowed to be applied at these positions. The accumulative depth based strategy is described in algorithm 5.3, where the pulse duration τ was not taken into account and set to a user defined constant.

Algorithm 5.3: Accumulative depth-based strategy [Kah09]

Input: Depth profile $D_{M\times N}$, critical point set P, channel radius R and laser beam radius r

Output: Ablation pattern $AP = \{(x_i, y_i; \tau \equiv \text{constant})\}$

1 $(x_c, y_c) \leftarrow$ coordinate of channel centre and *pattern* $\leftarrow \emptyset$

2 initialize all elements of flag matrix $F_{M\times N}$ false

3 set all $F(x, y)$ with $|(x, y) - (x_c, y_c)| < R - r$ true

4 **for** *all* $(x, y) \in P$ **do** `// eliminate critical points`

5   set all $F(x', y')$ with $|(x', y') - (x, y)| < r$ false

6 **while** *still exist* $F(x, y) = $ *true* **do**

7   locate (x_m, y_m) with the minimal $AD(x, y)$ among all still valid candidate points

8   append $(x_m, y_m; \tau)$ to AP

9   set all $F(x', y')$ with $|(x', y') - (x_m, y_m)| < 2r$ false

10 **return**

The command line 3 of algorithm 5.3 means that only the positions within the channel are valid candidates. Considering the non-zero beam radius r, the pulse centres have to further hold the distance r to the channel boundary, so that the complete pulse can be located inside the channel. For the same reason, the critical point set P is also expanded for r (command line 5), as illustrated in figure 5.28b.

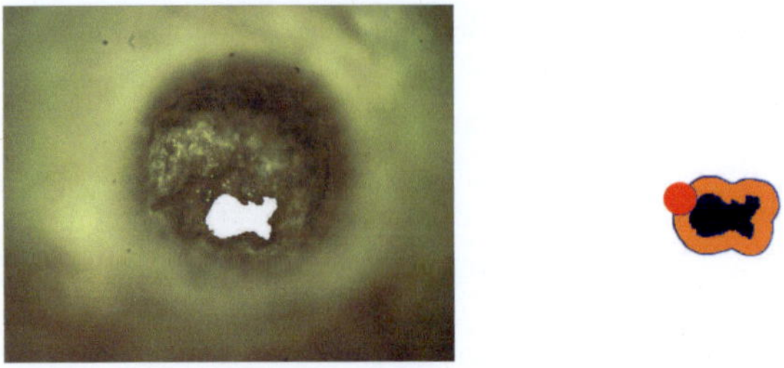

(a) (b)

Figure 5.28: (a) Critical point set P (white) denoting the region where the cochlear endosteum is already exposed to air or perforated in camera image; (b) expansion (orange region) of critical point set P for the laser beam radius r to ensure no pulse will overlap with the critical region (black). The red dot denotes the diameter of a laser spot. [Kah09]

After initializing the map of valid candidate positions, the pulse distribution is planned iteratively until no more valid position is remaining. During each loop, the position with the minimal accumulative depth is chosen for the next pulse, indicating the region covered by the laser pulse centred at this position has the minimal average depth within the whole channel. In other words, the chosen position is the shallowest region on the channel bottom. It is hence reasonable to apply the next pulse here. Moreover, if two pulses are overlapping, the depth profile within the overlapped part will already be changed by the first pulse, so that the decision made for the second one based on the original depth profile is no more valid. Therefore, no overlapping is allowed in an ablation pattern. As soon as a candidate is chosen, all positions within the radius of $2r$ to it are set to false (command line 9), so that any two pulses will be maximal tangent to each other.

Prediction of Post-Ablation Channel Shape Among the input parameters of algorithm 5.3, the current channel depth profile $D_{M\times N}$ and the critical point set P are unknown. While P can be determined from the camera images (figure 5.28a), no three-dimensional surface profile can be extracted from them directly.

Kahrs et al. and Burgner et al. [Kah09, Bur10] have therefore developed an additive model for predicting the channel shape after each round of ablation. With the help of a confocal microscope, the shape of the craters ablated by single laser pulses can be modelled (figure 5.29a-b).

Depending on varying pulse duration τ, the radius and depth of the crater model are different. The longer the pulse is, the deeper and larger will the resulting crater be.

The change of the surface profile at the channel bottom after applying the pulses in AP can be simply simulated by adding the corresponding single pulse model to each position (x_i, y_i) (figure 5.29c). Supposing the initial target tissue surface to be approximately flat, the current channel shape can be predicted by repeating this procedure round for round.

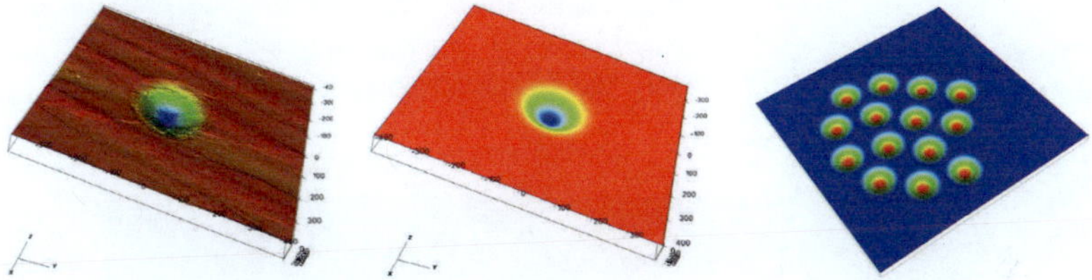

(a) (b) (c)

Figure 5.29: (a-b) Modelling of craters ablated by single laser pulses: (a) the 3D surface profile of the crater measured using a confocal microscope. (b) Approximation of the profile with a 2D Gaussian function. (c) Change of the channel shape profile after each round of ablation predicted by means of adding the single crater model (b) to the positions in the ablation pattern AP. [Kah09]

5.4.2 Residual Bone Thickness-based Strategy

Compared to the situation of Kahrs et al., the residual bone thickness distribution above the endosteum is now available, which can be used to guide the laser ablation. In this section, the algorithm 5.3 will be modified in order to take full advantage of this online measured information.

Determination of Pulse Position The residual bone thickness in the region of interest can be simply calculated by

$$T(x, y) = S(x, y) - M(x, y) - t_{\text{pre}} \tag{5.18}$$

where $S(x, y)$ and $M(x, y)$ are the positions of the bone surface and endosteum at (x, y) respectively. The user specified constant t_{pre} defines the thickness of a tissue layer to be preserved above the critical structure, whose value can be set arbitrarily and changed at any time during the ablation process. With this parameter, the surgeon is able to handle each patient individually regarding the different thickness of the endosteal layer. The surgeon may even preserve a thin bone layer above the critical structure as a physical protection of it until the final moment before inserting the implant. The corresponding critical point set P required by the algorithm 5.3 is then defined as

$$P = \{(x, y)|T(x, y) \leq 0\}$$

Accordingly, no more pulses are allowed to be shot to (x, y) if the local channel bottom at this position reaches the tissue layer to be preserved. Therefore, t_{pre} actually defines the "stop surface" of the laser ablation, as plotted in figure 5.30.

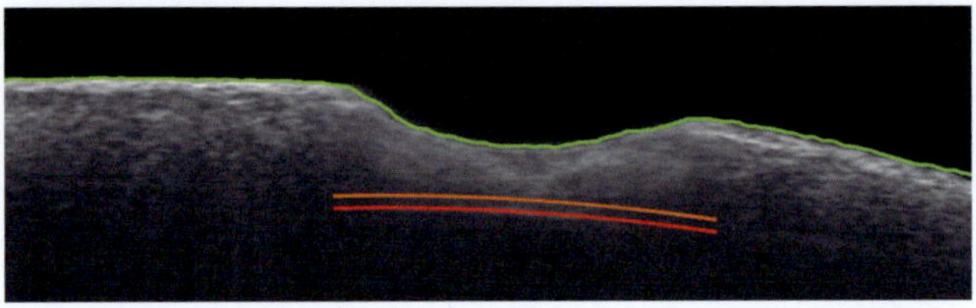

Figure 5.30: The position of bone surface (green), endosteum (red) and the tissue layer to be preserved (orange) within the volume of interest. The orange curve also defines the "stop surface" of the laser ablation.

The key step of the algorithm 5.3 is the command line 7, which determines the position of the next laser pulse. Knowing the current residual bone thickness distribution, we designed two different criteria $c(x, y)$ for finding the optimal pulse position. The first one is directly adapted from equation (5.17), where the channel depth profile is replaced by the residual bone thickness profile $T(x, y)$ defined by equation (5.18), yielding the *accumulative thickness*

$$c(x_0, y_0) = AT(x_0, y_0) = \sum_{|(x,y)-(x_0,y_0)|<r} T(x, y) \tag{5.19}$$

Meanwhile, $T(x, y)$ itself is chosen as the second version of the criterion

$$c(x_0, y_0) = T(x_0, y_0) \tag{5.20}$$

Correspondingly, instead of locating the position with minimal accumulative depth, the next pulse is planned to be applied to the position with the maximal $c(x, y)$. Thus, the positions of each pulse (x_i, y_i) in the ablation pattern $AP = \{(x_i, y_i; \tau_i)\}$ can be determined.

Determination of Pulse Duration In order to ensure the safety of the critical structure and simultaneously make the resulting channel bottom as smooth as possible, the pulse duration τ_i is also taken into account. A trivial idea is to apply longer pulses to the places where the residual bone tissue is thicker and shorter ones to the thinner places.

For the sake of simplicity in laser control and crater modelling, only three pulse durations $\{20, 40, 60\}$ μs are set as candidates for τ_i, providing a discrimination of 15-20 μm between different choices. The craters ablated by these pulses are modelled using the method proposed by Kahrs and Burgner et al. introduced in figure 5.29a-b. For any planned pulse position (x_i, y_i) and a candidate pulse duration $\tau \in \{20, 40, 60\}$ μs , the minimal residual bone thickness within the laser spot after applying the pulse can be predicted accordingly, which are appended to a list $\{RT_{i\tau}^{\min}\}$. All candidate pulses in this list have to pass two checks.

First, a so called *safety check* is performed. Obviously, a negative $RT_{i\tau}^{\min}$ indicates that the candidate pulse $(x_i, y_i; \tau)$ has penetrated the "stop surface". Therefore, all such candidate pulses are eliminated from $\{RT_{i\tau}^{\min}\}$ to avoid potential injury to the critical structure foresightedly, which is the major purpose of this work. Particularly, an empty $\{RT_{i\tau}^{\min}\}$ after trying all possible pulse positions indicates that the "stop surface" has been overall reached.

In addition, a *roughness check* is developed in order to prevent the formation of "islands" on the bottom of the resulting channel (figure 5.31a). Due to the gaussian-shaped craters (figure 5.29a-b), it is impossible to ablate a perfectly smooth surface. As a result, peaks and valleys are unavoidable on the resulting channel bottom. While the valley bottom already touches the "stop surface", there often remains a thick layer of bone tissue on the neighbouring peaks.

According to the criteria (5.19) or (5.20), a spontaneous action is to apply a pulse to these peaks (figure 5.31a). However, the peaks are in many cases so narrow, that the margin of the pulse overlaps the valley, resulting in a negative $RT_{i\tau}^{\min}$. The candidate position hence fails to pass the safety check. Consequently, these peaks will never be ablated by any succeeding laser pulses and remain on the channel bottom.

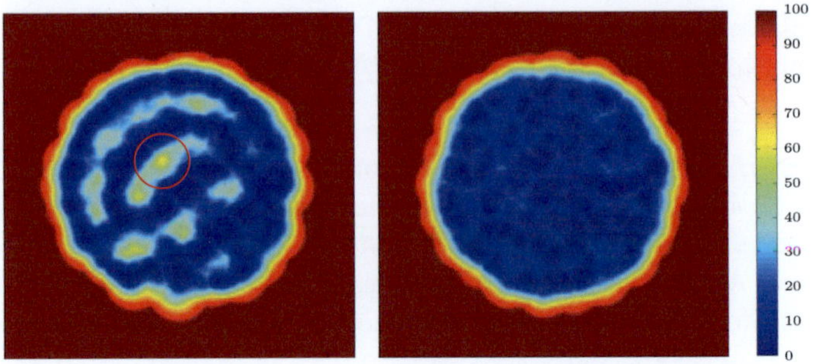

(a) (b)

Figure 5.31: Simulated residual bone thickness distribution after termination of the laser ablation (a) without and (b) with roughness check under the same initial condition. The pulse planned at the marked position in (a) is eliminated due to the risk of penetrating the "stop surface" at its upper-left and right-bottom corners (failure by safety check). Unit: voxels.

Considering that the formation of peaks and valleys is inevitable, the only choice is to limit the thickness difference between them. For this purpose, the roughness check is performed as follows: first, the average of the remaining elements in $\{RT_{i\tau}^{\min}\}$ is calculated, noted as $\overline{RT}$. An empirical threshold τ_{60} indicating the average ablation depth of a 60 μs pulse is set. If a candidate pulse $(x_i, y_i; \tau)$ satisfies $\overline{RT} - RT_{i\tau}^{\min} > \tau_{60}$, it will potentially cause a valley much deeper than the average level on the whole channel bottom. All such pulses are removed from the list $\{RT_{i\tau}^{\min}\}$ to ensure a uniformly distributed residual bone thickness.

If all three candidate pulse durations of a position (x_i, y_i) have been eliminated from $\{RT_{i\tau}^{\min}\}$, this position will be removed from the ablation pattern AP. On the other hand, if more than one candidate τ have passed both safety and roughness checks, the longest τ will be chosen, so that a relatively higher ablation efficiency can be achieved. Thus, the residual bone thickness will be uniformly decreased on the channel bottom without forming deep valleys. No high peaks will occur on the channel bottom while the ablation process is terminated (figure 5.31b).

Moreover, the ablation pattern is extended to three-dimensional as a 4-tuple $AP = \{(x_i, y_i, z_i; \tau_i)\}$, where $z_i = S(x_i, y_i)$ denotes the corresponding surface position before applying the planned pulse to (x_i, y_i). With the increasing channel depth, the channel bottom may exceed the Rayleigh range of the OCT or the CO_2 laser in the vertical direction. In such a case, the enlarged working distance between the channel bottom and the laser optics can be compensated using a robot (see also setup in figure 6.1b) to ensure the best imaging and ablation quality. The whole planning procedure is summarised in algorithm 5.4.

Algorithm 5.4: Residual bone thickness-based ablation strategy

Input: Thickness profile $T_{M\times N}$, surface profile $S_{M\times N}$, critical point set P, channel radius R and laser beam radius r
Output: Ablation pattern $AP = \{(x_i, y_i, z_i; \tau_i)\}$

$(x_c, y_c) \leftarrow$ coordinate of channel centre
$AP \leftarrow \emptyset$ and $\{RT_{i\tau}^{\min}\} \leftarrow \emptyset$
initialize all elements of flag matrix $F_{M\times N}$ false
set all $F(x, y)$ with $|(x, y) - (x_c, y_c)| < R - r$ true
for *all* $(x, y) \in P$ **do** // eliminate critical points
    set all $F(x', y')$ with $|(x', y') - (x, y)| < r$ false
while *still exist* $F(x, y) = true$ **do**
    locate (x_m, y_m) with the maximal $c(x, y)$ among all still valid candidates, $c(x, y)$ chooses either equation (5.19) or (5.20)
    append $(x_m, y_m, S(x_m, y_m); \tau)$ to AP with $\tau \in \{20, 40, 60\}\,\mu s$ undetermined yet
    $i \leftarrow$ the number of pulses in AP
    calculate $RT_{i\tau}^{\min}$ for all three candidate τ
    if *all three* $RT_{i\tau}^{\min} < 0$ **then** // safety check
        eliminate $(x_m, y_m, S(x_m, y_m); \tau)$ from AP
        $F(x_m, y_m) \leftarrow$ false
    else
        append all positive $RT_{i\tau}^{\min}$ to $\{RT_{i\tau}^{\min}\}$
        set all $F(x', y')$ with $|(x', y') - (x_m, y_m)| < 2r$ false
$\overline{RT} \leftarrow$ average of $\{RT_{i\tau}^{\min}\}$
eliminate all $RT_{i\tau}^{\min} < \overline{RT} - \tau_{60}$ from $\{RT_{i\tau}^{\min}\}$// roughness check
for *all* $(x_i, y_i, z_i; \tau_i) \in AP$ **do** // determine pulse duration
    if *all three* $RT_{i\tau}^{\min}$ *have been eliminated* **then**
        eliminate $(x_i, y_i, z_i; \tau_i)$ from AP
    else
        $\tau_i \leftarrow$ the longest τ whose $RT_{i\tau}^{\min}$ has passed roughness checks
return

Pre- and Post-Segmentation Phases Noticing that the endosteum is completely invisible while the overlying bone tissue is very thick (for example figure 5.5b). Only when the thickness is reduced to about 500 μm, the segmentation of the endosteum can be performed.

The planning is hence divided into two phases, namely pre- and post-segmentation phases[8]. For the pre-segmentation phase, a virtual endosteum is set to be at a depth of infinity and parallel to the original bone surface, resulting in uniformly distributed pulses with the maximal possible pulse duration. Once the endosteum is detected, the system is switched to the post-segmentation phase. The ablation pattern is then planned according to the online measured residual bone thickness and start to approach the shape of the critical structure automatically.

The ablation terminates when the resulting $AP = \emptyset$, indicating that the tissue layer to be preserved is reached. Figure 5.32 shows examples of the planning according to algorithm 5.4 during the pre- and post-segmentation phases. As expected, the pulses are assigned to the positions with thicker residual bone layer (sub-figure a). Meanwhile, the pulse durations are automatically adjusted according to the thickness distribution (sub-figure b).

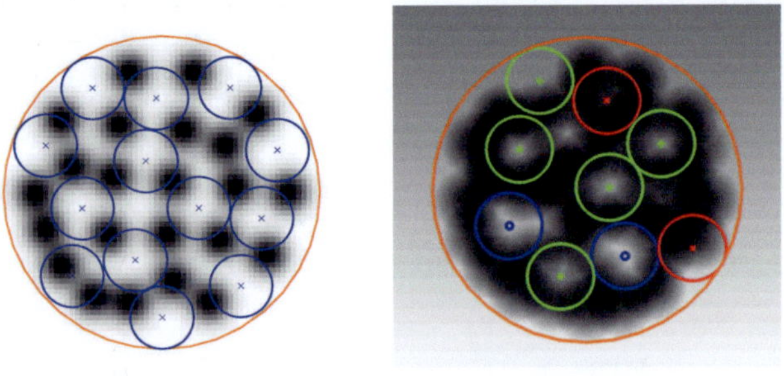

(a) (b)

Figure 5.32: (a-b) Examples of the resulting ablation pattern calculated using algorithm 5.4, where the red, green and blue circles denote the positions of fine, mild and rough pulses respectively while the large orange circle is the channel boundary. The gray scale in the background indicates the thickness of the residual bone tissue where darker pixels denote a lower thickness and vice versa: (a) pre-segmentation phase; (b)post-segmentation phase.

[8] Effect of these two phases see figure 6.15a.

5.5 Summary

In this chapter, the artefacts in the OCT scans hindering the correct detection of the cochlear endosteum, namely stripe noises, fan distortion and uncompensated refractive index, are analysed in detail. Corresponding correction methods are developed. Without requiring special equipments, an ingenious method using OCT itself for measuring the refractive index of the bony shell of cochlea is proposed, which can be applied not only pre-operatively, but also intra-operatively for each patient individually. A novel speckle noise reduction technique with high effectiveness and low computational cost is invented, which can significantly improve the quality of the OCT images. The workflow of detecting the cochlear endosteum in the enhanced OCT volumes is then designed. According to the resulting residual bone thickness profile, a strategy for planning the pulse positions and pulse durations is proposed, which approaches the shape of the cochlear endosteum and meanwhile prevents injuries to this fragile structure.

The key issue of establishing a closed-loop control of laser-cochleostomy is thereby successfully solved.

CHAPTER 6

System Integration and Evaluation

So far, the most important part of the control loop proposed in figure 3.10, from OCT scanning to ablation planning, has been successfully established. The next scientific challenge is now: how to integrate the OCT and CO_2 laser ablation systems, so that the ablation pattern planned in the OCT scans can be precisely executed by the CO_2 laser?

In this chapter, a bridge connecting these two cutting-edge technologies will be built. First, a coaxial setup for physically combining both systems is realised. Then, an innovative patient tracking mechanism using OCT itself is proposed, so that the relative movements between the patient and the lasers can be compensated. After that, a three dimensional mapping between the workspaces of the OCT and CO_2 laser is determined, enabling a precise coordinate transformation between both scanning optics. The control loop of the laser-cochleostomy using OCT is thereby completed and the whole system is experimentally evaluated.

6.1 Coaxial Setup of OCT and CO_2 Laser

Before being able to coordinate with each other, the OCT and the CO_2 laser have to be physically brought together, so that their working space (see figure 2.8) are overlapped and the ablation area of the CO_2 laser can be monitored by the OCT. For this purpose, a coaxial setup combining the both systems is designed, as illustrated in figure 6.1a.

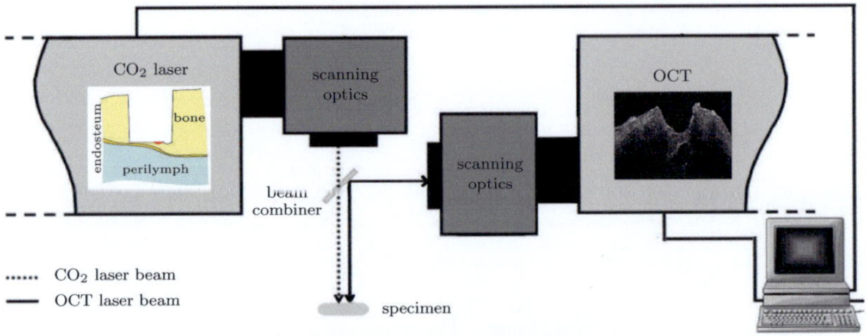

(a)

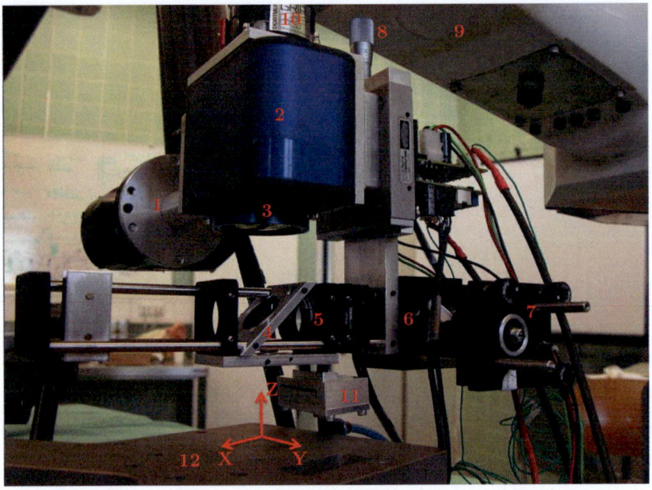

(b)

Figure 6.1: (a) Schematic diagram of the coaxial setup[1] combining the OCT and the CO_2 laser systems together. (b) Physical realisation of the setup: 1. CO_2 laser input; 2. CO_2 laser scanner; 3. CO_2 laser focusing lens; 4. beam combiner; 5. OCT focusing lens; 6. OCT scanner; 7. OCT laser input; 8. z-positioning screw; 9. robot arm; 10. robot flange; 11. air spray; 12. platform of hexapod and its coordinate system.

The ablating CO_2 laser beam is oriented vertically downwards while the measuring beam of the OCT comes from the horizontal direction. The key component of this setup is the beam combiner, which is a dichroic germanium mirror with high reflectivity coating for the wave-

[1] The author appreciates the project partners from the chair for BioMolecular Optics at the University of Munich, Germany for designing and realizing this setup.

lengths around 1.3 μm. The beam combiner is therefore transparent for the wavelength of the CO_2 laser (10.6 μm) while reflecting the wavelength of the OCT measuring beam (1310±50 nm). The mirror is installed 45° to the vertical direction, so that the horizontally incident OCT measuring beam is exactly deflected for 90° and turns vertically downwards, while the CO_2 laser beam passes through the transparent mirror and keeps its original direction. Thus, the optical axes of both systems are overlapped with each other below the beam combiner, so that their working space will cover the same area.

Figure 6.1b shows the physical realisation of the coaxial setup, where the z-positioning screw is used to adjust the vertical position of the beam combiner and OCT scanning optics (4-7) relative to the CO_2 laser optics (1-3), in order to align their beam waists (focal planes) together. The workspaces of both systems are thereby overlapped in all three dimensions. After the adjustment, the z-position screw is fixed to ensure a rigid connection between the two systems. This optics complex is fixed to a robot arm for a precise positioning to the desired location. In the following, this complex consisting of both scanning optics will be referred to as the *OCT-CO_2 optics*.

An extra horizontal air spray supplied with pressure air is installed below the beam combiner to blow the ablation debris away and thus prevent smearing of the optics. In addition, a hexapod M-850 (Physik Instrumente GmbH & Co. KG, Karlsruhe, Germany) with high positioning precision is used as a reference system for the accuracy evaluation in the following sections. The relevant specifications are summarised in table 6.1, where the U, V, W are rotations about the X, Y, Z axes respectively.

Table 6.1: Relevant technical specifications of the 6-DOF M-850 hexapod, which is used as a highly accurate reference positioning system in the following sections [Phy03].

property	value	property	value
Travel X, Y	±50 mm	Travel U, V	±15 deg
Repeatability X, Y	±2 μm	Repeatability U, V	±10 μrad
Travel Z	±25 mm	Travel W	±30 deg
Repeatability Z	±1 μm	Repeatability W	±10 μrad

6.2 Patient Tracking using OCT

6.2.1 Motivation

Working with extremely high precision, OCT guided laser-cochleostomy system is very sensitive to relative movements between the patient and the OCT-CO_2 optics. Considering the tiny diameter of the CO_2 laser pulses which is only approximately 200 μm, even tiny displacements less than 100 μm can let the pulses be shot to wrong positions and make the best ablation planning pointless. In worst case, erroneously applied pulses can damage the endosteum instantly if parts of it are already exposed (figure 6.2a-b).

Unfortunately, such movements are almost unavoidable, even under laboratory condition. Figure 6.2c shows a case during an ablation experiment, where the personnel happened to lean against the 250 kg heavy measuring table to supervise the ablation, resulting in a relative translation of about 300 μm. The pulses originally planned to be applied to the channel bottom were erroneously shot to the lip on the right. It would be critical if this happened in real operation room where no heavy measuring table is available. Physical contacts to the patient, to the OP-table or to the OCT-CO_2 optics can lead to such a movement on hundred micrometer scale.

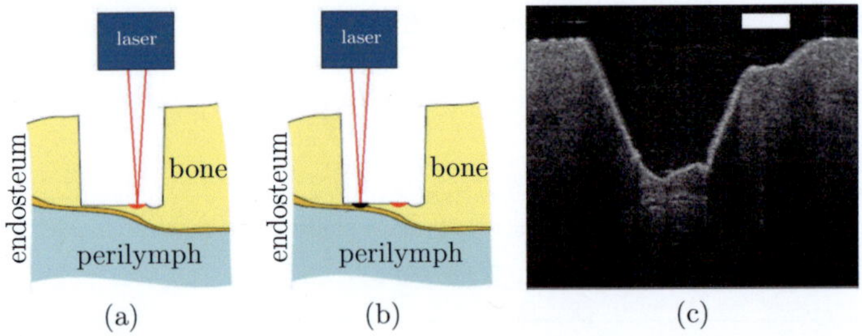

Figure 6.2: (a-b) Illustration of a critical situation induced by relative movement between the patient and OCT-CO_2 optics: (a) planned position and (b) pulse applied to the endosteum due to the movement. (c) An example of erroneously applied pulses, resulting in the stair-shaped structure at the channel lip, bar=250 μm.

For the sake of patients' safety, motion compensation for such movements is mandatory and an accuracy less than 50 μm is desired considering the small size of the laser pulses. In the context of computer-assisted surgery (CAS), optical or electromagnetic tracking systems are considered to be the gold standard for this purpose and have already been widely used since years [RPS+08, LCG+08, MSRW10, MHTG+11, vJZZG13]. Special trackers, e.g. rigid bodies with retro-reflective marker spheres (figure 6.3a) or electromagnetic tracking coils, are attached to the object to be tracked. Figure 6.3b illustrates a typical setup of using such a tracking system to perform the motion compensation between the patient and the laser optics in our case.

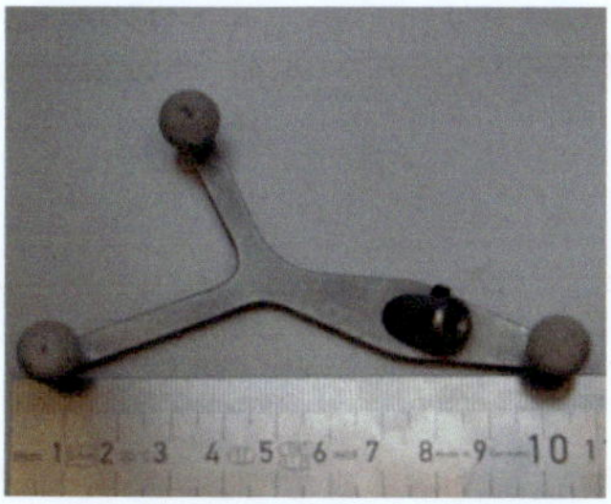

(a)

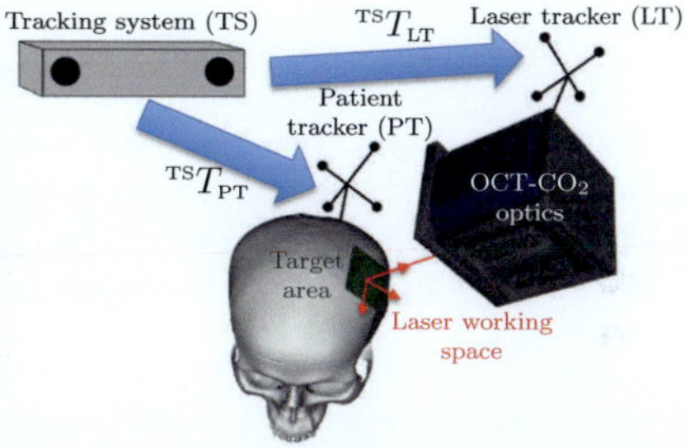

(b)

Figure 6.3: (a) A typical rigid body with three marker spheres. (b) Illustration of a typical setup of using a conventional tracking system to perform the motion compensation, where special trackers are attached to the patient and the laser optics respectively. The position and orientation of the trackers are monitored by the tracking system. Based on this information, the relative movements between the target area and the laser working space are determined indirectly.

The location and orientation of the trackers ($^{TS}T_{LT}$ and $^{TS}T_{PT}$) are delivered by the tracking system in real time, which are 4×4 homogeneous matrices. The movements between the target area and the laser working space can be detected by monitoring the transformation from the the laser tracker to the patient tracker:

$$^{LT}T_{PT} = ^{TS}T_{LT}^{-1} \cdot ^{TS}T_{PT} \tag{6.1}$$

However, the tracking accuracy of most commercially available tracking systems ranges from several hundred micrometers to one millimetre. The state of the art NDI Polaris optical tracking system for example, provides a measuring accuracy of 0.25-0.35 mm (RMS, root mean square) per tracked rigid body with a 95% confidence interval (CI) of 0.5-0.6 mm according to the official specification of the manufacturer. The electromagnetic tracking systems, e.g. the NDI Aurora, provide generally even poor performance of about 1 mm. An even lower accuracy of the resulting ${}^{\text{LT}}T_{\text{PT}}$ is expected while two trackers are used in our case (figure 6.3b) due to the accumulation of measuring errors in ${}^{\text{TS}}T_{\text{LT}}$ and ${}^{\text{TS}}T_{\text{PT}}$.

Moreover, what the tracking system measures is not the location of the region of interest (ROI) directly, e.g. the target area and the laser working space in our case, but the position and orientation of the attached trackers. Generally, the trackers have the diagonal size of 5-10 cm (figure 6.3a) and are therefore difficult to be attached to the target area directly, especially in the case of cochleostomy whose diameter is only circa 1 mm. Neither can they be fixed to the laser working space in front of the optics. Consequently, registration between the target area and the patient tracker as well as between the laser working space and the laser tracker has to be performed. The unavoidable registration errors will however introduce extra inaccuracy to the tracking result.

Meanwhile, the distance between the tracker and the ROI also magnifies the rotational error of the tracking system. For example, the distance between the laser working space and the laser optics that is larger than 11 cm in our setup, which is also corresponding to the distance from the laser tracker to the laser working space. At such a distance, even a slight rotational tracking error of 0.1° can already lead to an extra translational error of about 200 μm in addition to the error sources stated above.

As a result, the global tracking accuracy of the tool tip (corresponding to the center of the laser working space in our case) with respect to the target using similar setup in figure 6.3b generally ranges from 0.5 mm to even more than 1 mm [RPS+08, LCG+08, MSRW10, MHTG+11, vJZZG13], which is obviously insufficient for our case.

Reviewing the shortcomings of the conventional tracking system stated above, it can be concluded that the main reason for the relatively low tracking accuracy is caused by the following factors:

- Insufficient tracking accuracy of each single tracker
- Complicated transformation chain from target area to the laser working space due to indirect tracking: target area → patient tracker → tracking system → laser tracker → laser working space
- Rotational tracking error magnified by the distance between the trackers and ROI

Noticing that the in laser-ablation system integrated OCT itself can "see" the target area directly and provides a high resolution on micrometer scale, a spontaneous idea is: why not use the OCT itself as an optical tracking system?

6.2.2 OCT as Tracking System

6.2.2.1 Tracking Concept

Eilers et. al. [EWO+09] have already proposed a highly accurate multimodal registration method between OCT and flat panel volume computerised tomography (fpVCT) based on comparing the internal structures of the scanned volume. In theory, the tracking during the laser-cochleostomy can be realised by the registration of two successive OCT volumes applying this method.

However, from the divers OCT scans of the cochlea shown in the previous chapters it can be concluded that there exist very few internal structures inside the cochlea except small part of the scalae, which are invisible while the overlying bone tissue is thick. Therefore, it would be almost impossible to align two scans together based on analysing the internal structures of the cochlea. Moreover, comparing the whole 3D volume requires a high computational cost. It is hence difficult to achieve an acceptable tracking speed. Consequently, the internal structure based tracking is in principle not practical.

On the other hand, the experience from section 5.1.3.3 reveals that the sample surface is always very clear and easy to be detected in OCT scans. Therefore, the basic idea is: only make use of the 2D terrain information of the target surface obtained from the OCT scan instead of comparing the whole 3D volume. For a more stable and more efficient tracking, artificial landmarks are ablated using the CO_2 laser around the cochleostomy before starting the ablation process. By means of locating these landmarks, the position and orientation of the sample relative to the OCT-CO_2 optics can be obtained.

Preliminary feasibility study for this tracking concept was conducted on a formalin fixed human cochlea. Three landmarks were drilled asymmetrically arround the cochleostomy, as shown in figure 6.4a.

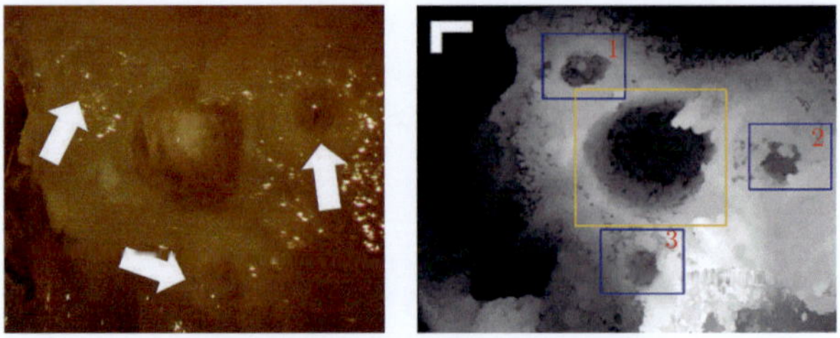

(a) (b)

Figure 6.4: Feasibility study of the proposed tracking concept: (a) microscopic photo of the artificial landmarks drilled with diamond burr surrounding the cochleostomy on a human cochlea; (b) the corresponding surface profile extracted from the OCT scan, where the yellow grid denotes the volume of interest and the blue grids 1-3 are the search regions of the corresponding landmarks, bar=500 μm.

While choosing the appropriate positions and sizes of the landmarks, the following criteria have to be satisfied:

i. No critical structures are injured.

ii. The size of the landmarks is sufficiently large to be distinguished from natural structures on the original surface.

iii. The landmarks are located as far as possible to each other.

iv. The macroscopic curvature of the original surface should not be very large, i.e. relatively flat.

The criteria iii and iv can make the detection of the landmarks easier (refer to section 6.2.2.2). The criterion iii also serves to increase the rotational tracking accuracy.

As stated in the motivation, the purpose of the proposed tracking concept is to supplement the conventional tracking system to detect the tiny movements between the patient and OCT-CO_2 optics ranging from tens of micrometers to several hundred micrometers, i.e. the translation of each landmark is limited to a small range. Therefore, knowing the landmark positions in the previous scan, small search regions centred at these positions can be defined in the subsequent one (figure 6.4b). The size of the search regions is recommended to be 0.5-1 mm according to the environment. For a more efficient tracking, only the A-scans within the chosen search regions will be processed during the tracking loop. Each tracking loop is divided into two steps: single landmark detection and fiducial registration, as introduced in the following two sections.

6.2.2.2 Single Landmark Detection

As the first step, the accurate position of each single landmark has to be detected within the given search region, which is defined as the centroid of all the surface vertices within its boundary on the bone surface. Due to the criterion iii of the tracking concept, it can be further guaranteed that there exists exactly one landmark within each search region. In the following, the search region 3 of figure 6.4b is taken as an example to explain the workflow of the detection.

As described in section 3.1.1, the axial and spatial pixel sizes are independent from each other, i.e. the pixel size in x and y directions is generally different as the z direction. Therefore, the very first step is to compensate this difference to ensure the unit vectors in all three directions have the same length.

The basic idea of the detection is to regard the surface profile within the search regions as gray value image, so that the conventional boundary detection and pattern recognition techniques can be applied directly. Observing the cross-sectional image of the landmark shown in figure 6.5a, it can be affirmed that landmarks are sunken structures with negative second order derivative on its boundary. The standard method for extracting the second order derivative is to apply the Gaussian operator first and then the Laplace operator (refer to section 4.1) to the image respectively. Despite the Gaussian operator, the second order derivative is still sensible to noises. Gonzalez et al. have hence suggested to multiply the first and second order derivatives together to emphasis the real boundaries [GW02].

The first order derivatives can be obtained with the Sobel operators (equation (4.4)) and the histogram based thresholding (refer to figure 5.4b and relevant texts) is applied to the product of the first and the second order derivatives to eliminate non-candidate pixels. The result of applying the above procedure to the search region 3 is shown in figure 6.5b, where the quasi circular landmark boundary can be recognized while a lot of noisy structures are also visible outside the landmark boundary[2]. Noticing that the landmarks are artificially generated, their radius can be roughly estimated, supposing to be r.

[2] The reason for these noises is that the cochleostomy and landmarks were drilled with a diamond burr, so that the sample surface is randomly covered by some tiny milling debris, which can be discovered near the landmark boundary in figure 6.5a if observed more closely. The noisy curves are the contours of the debris.

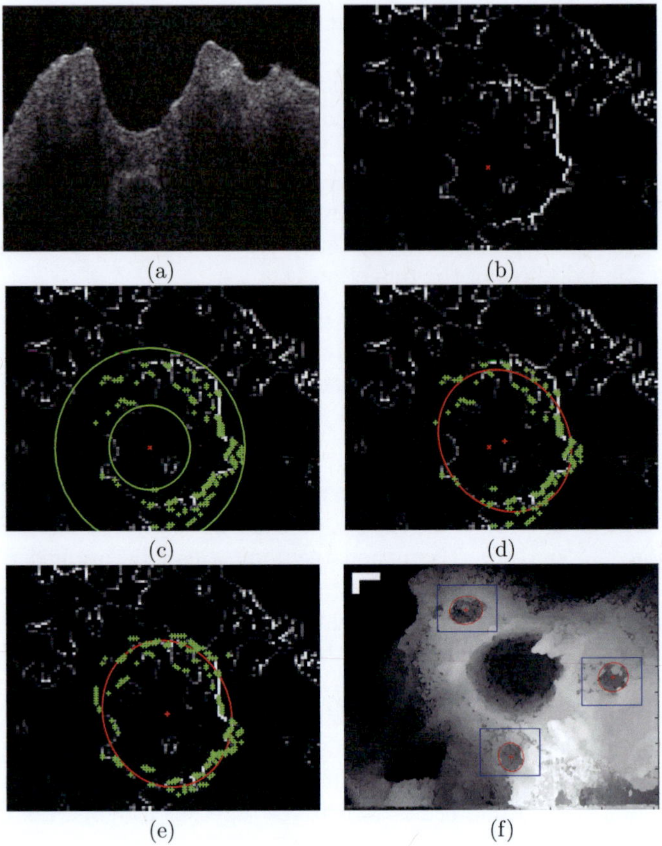

Figure 6.5: (a) An example OCT image passing through the cochleostomy with a landmark on its right side. (b-e) Workflow of landmark detection taking the search region 3 in figure 6.4b as example: (b) the candidate boundary pixels and the landmark centre (red x) estimated using cross-correlation with a circular pattern; (c) the tolerance range (between the green circles) and the valid candidate boundary pixels (green +) after gradient examination; (d) the ellipse fit to the valid candidate boundary pixels and the resulting new landmark centre (red +); (e) the detected landmark boundary and its centre after termination of the algorithm. (f) The results of landmark detection applied to figure 6.4b, bar=500 μm.

A common method to estimate the centre of such a quasi circular object with known radius is to calculate its cross-correlation with a circular pattern having the same radius and then search for the position with the maximal coefficient [Tre10]. The discrete cross-correlation can be calculated using equation (4.2) and the resulting position is marked with a red x in figure 6.5b.

However, due to the milling debris, the landmark boundary is actually not regular. Moreover, the landmark itself might also be elliptical rather than circular (e.g. the landmark in search region 1) and the landmark radius r is also roughly estimated. Consequently, the cross-correlation based procedure can only give a rough estimation of the landmark centre and a subsequent correction is hence necessary. For this purpose, a ring-shaped tolerance range surrounding the estimated centre is defined, as shown in figure 6.5c. All candidates outside this range are regarded as invalid. Moreover, a gradient examination is performed for every remaining candidate pixel P. Suppose the estimated landmark centre is C and the surface gradient at P is ∇P. It can be intuitively inferred that ∇P at any point on the landmark boundary should be roughly pointing to the landmark centre due to the shape of the landmark. Hence, the angle between ∇P and the vector $\vec{PC}$ is not allowed to exceed a predefined value for a valid candidate. Empirically, the ring-shaped tolerance range is set to the size of $0.6r$-$1.25r$ and the threshold for the gradient examination is chosen as $\pm\pi/6$.

The resulting candidate boundary pixels are plotted in figure 6.5c with green crosses. An ellipse is then obtained using least squares fitting to these pixels and the ellipse centre is regarded as the new estimation of the landmark centre, as plotted in sub-figure d. Repeating the procedure of defining tolerance range, gradient examination and ellipse fitting until the change of the estimated centre position between two iterations is smaller than a given stopping criterion or the maximal iteration number is reached, the workflow terminates. The resulting ellipse is then regarded as the landmark boundary (sub-figure e). Each surface vertex within this ellipse is given a weight based on the area of its adjacent surface polygons and the centroid can be then intuitively calculated. Algorithm 6.1 summarises the workflow above.

Empirically, the stopping criterion is set to 1/4 pixel and the maximal iteration number is set to 20. The figure 6.5f shows the results of applying algorithm 6.1 to all three search regions in figure 6.4b. It can be observed that all three landmarks are precisely located on macroscopic scale. This also evidences the robustness of the algorithm in the case that the landmarks are partially covered by the milling debris, resulting in irregular shape of the landmark boundaries, especially in the search region 2. By means of defining the tolerance range, gradient examination and the ellipse fitting, the approach is able to recover the boundary according to the remaining visible part. In general, the maximal number of iterations[3] would be exceeded only when a wrong radius estimation r with too large deviation from the actual value is given, or the most part of the landmark is covered by milling debris. An anew radius estimation or cleaning the landmarks can solve the problem accordingly.

Algorithm 6.1: Landmark detection within a given search region.

Input: Surface profile of the search region as an image I, rough estimation of the landmark radius r, stopping criterion SC

Output: Centroid C

Compensate pixel size difference between spatial and lateral directions

$M \leftarrow |I'.*I''|$ `// element-wise multiplication of derivatives`

set all elements of M having positive 2nd order derivatives to zero

histogram based thresholding of M and $T \leftarrow$ obtained threshold

$CP \leftarrow$ circular pattern with radius r

$X \leftarrow M * CP$ `// cross-correlation`

$C_{est} \leftarrow$ position of the maximal element in X

$\Delta \leftarrow \infty$

while $\Delta > SC$ *or maximal iteration number not reached* **do**

- define tolerance range surrounding C_{est}
- $S \leftarrow$ all candidate pixels with $M > T$ within tolerance range
- perform gradient examination to S
- $E \leftarrow$ least squares ellipse fitting to remaining pixels in S
- $C'_{est} \leftarrow C_{est}$ and $C_{est} \leftarrow$ centre of E
- $\Delta \leftarrow |C'_{est} - C_{est}|$

$C \leftarrow$ centroid of all vertices within E

return

6.2.2.3 Fiducial Registration

Knowing the positions of each single landmark, the relative movement of the target sample between two OCT scans acquired at different time

[3] See also the evaluations in section 6.2.3.1 where an average number of the iterations is given.

point can then be calculated accordingly. Obviously, once the landmarks are ablated on the bone surface, their geometric layout is fixed, spanning a "rigid body" similar to the conventional optical tracking system (see figure 6.3). Knowing the position of each single landmark, the tracking of the target movement in such a case is a mature technology, known as *point based rigid registration*, which will be briefly introduced in the following. More details of this technology can be found in [FS00].

Suppose N landmarks are used where $N \geq 3$ and denote their 3D positions in the previous and current OCT scans as $\mathbf{x}_i$ and $\mathbf{y}_i$ ($i = 1 \cdots N$) respectively. Then the relative movement of the sample can be calculated by the following steps:

1. Compute the centroid of the fiducial configuration in each scan:

$$\bar{\mathbf{x}} = \frac{1}{N}\sum_{i=1}^{N}\mathbf{x}_i, \qquad \bar{\mathbf{y}} = \frac{1}{N}\sum_{i=1}^{N}\mathbf{y}_i$$

2. Compute the fiducial covariance matrix:

$$H = \sum_{i=1}^{N}(\mathbf{x}_i - \bar{\mathbf{x}})(\mathbf{y}_i - \bar{\mathbf{y}})$$

3. Perform singular value decomposition (SVD) of H:

$$H = U\Lambda V^t$$

   where $U^tU = V^tV = I$ and $\Lambda =$diag$(\lambda_1, \lambda_2, \lambda_3)$ that satisfy $\lambda_1 \geq \lambda_2 \geq \lambda_3 \geq 0$.

4. $R = V\mathrm{diag}(1, 1, \det(VU))\, U^t$.
5. $\mathbf{t} = \bar{\mathbf{y}} - R \cdot \bar{\mathbf{x}}$

The resulting R and $\mathbf{t}$ describe exactly the relative rotation and translation from the previous scan to the current one. Correspondingly, any point $\mathbf{p}_{\text{pre}} = (x, y, z)^t$ given in the previous scan will be located at the new position $\mathbf{p}_{\text{cur}}$ in the current one:

$$\mathbf{p}_{\text{cur}} = R \cdot \mathbf{p}_{\text{pre}} + \mathbf{t} \tag{6.2}$$

6.2.3 Experimental Evaluation

In order to quantitatively evaluate the accuracy of the proposed tracking mechanism, experiments were conducted for the single landmark detection as well as the complete tracking procedure with multiple landmarks, as reported in this section.

6.2.3.1 Single Landmark Detection

Considering that a pure translation of the landmark within a given search range only changes the position of all the candidate pixels for a same constant (see figure 6.5b), it will have no influence on the accuracy of the result. Contrarily, a rotation of the landmark will significantly affect the derivatives of the surface profile, based on which the landmark position is detected. Therefore, the experiments were designed to evaluate the accuracy of the algorithm under different incident angles. Moreover, considering that the aim of the tracking is to detect tiny movements of the patient, the test angles were further limited to 0-30°. Two groups of experiments were conducted with simulation data and real OCT data respectively.

For the first group, surface profiles of landmarks with different shapes (Gaussian and half sphere shaped) under divers incident angles were manually generated, whose centroids can be hence analytically calculated based on their geometry, which are regarded as reference results. Obviously, larger and deeper landmarks will be easier to detect. Therefore, while generating the simulation data, the dimension of the landmarks were chosen as small as possible, where the diameter and depth were set to 12 and 4 pixels respectively (figure 6.6)a.

For the second group, landmark craters were ablated with the CO_2 laser on bovine bone specimens. In order to generate reference centroids for the evaluation, square-shaped reference grids were also ablated surrounding the test landmarks (figure 6.6b). The landmarks were circa 125 μm deep with a diameter of about 200 μm and located exactly at the centre of the grid. Two specimens were prepared, one of them was manually polished with flat surface while the other one retains the original rough periosteum surface that is also slightly curved.

In order to make the result be comparable with the simulated landmarks of the first group, the scanning density of 50 A-scans per millimetre was while acquiring the OCT scans. The landmarks have hence the diameter of circa 10 pixels in the scans obtained. The four edges of the reference grid were detected with Hough transform [Hou62] in the surface profile extracted from the OCT scans (sub-figure c). The projection of the grid centre onto the original sample surface could be then calculated.

It should be noticed that the real centroid of the landmark does not lie on the original surface but some where inside the crater. The offset from the surface to the real centroid is hence estimated based on the crater models developed by Kahrs and Burgner et al. (refer to figure 5.29a-b and [Kah09, Bur10]). Subtract this offset from the grid centre obtained above along the surface normal, the reference centroids were obtained.

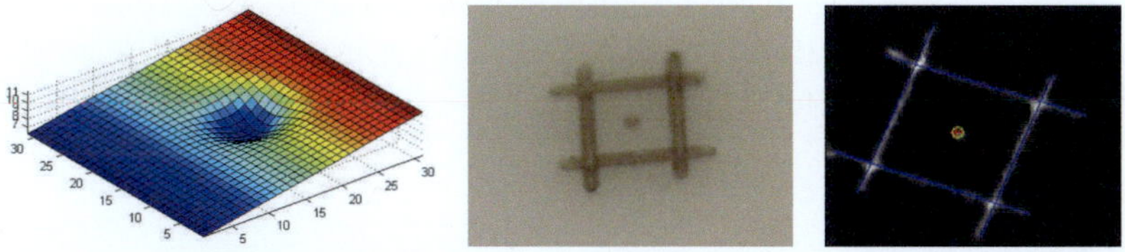

(a) (b) (c)

Figure 6.6: (a) A simulated Gaussian shaped test landmark under the incident angle of 10°; (b) a test landmark at the centre of a reference grid ablated on bovine bone specimen and (c) its surface profile in OCT scan with the centroid detected by algorithm 6.1 (red cross), the reference grid (blue lines) and corresponding reference centroid (yellow circle).

The absolute errors between the results of algorithm 6.1 and the reference centroids are listed in table 6.2, where the algorithm terminates after 2.89 iterations on average and maximal 5 iterations for all the test landmarks. Despite the small size of the landmarks which makes the detection more difficult, the mean absolute errors to the analytical reference centroids are only about half a voxel for the simulated landmarks. Due to the sharper landmark lip leading to larger second order derivatives, the half sphere shaped landmarks appear to have higher accuracy than the Gaussian shaped ones. For the real landmarks in the second group, the mean absolute error to the estimated reference centroids is around 30 μm. However, the roughness of the native periosteum surface does have negative influence on the detection accuracy. Nevertheless, the average error of 33.07 μm is still about ten times so accurate as the conventional marker based tracking system. No dependency of the errors on the incident angle can be concluded from either of the two groups.

Table 6.2: Absolute errors and mean absolute error (MAE) between the results of algorithm 6.1 and the reference centroids in three-dimensional space.

group	shape/surface	0°	5°	10°	15°	20°	25°	30°	MAE
I	Gaussian	0.73	0.73	0.81	0.62	0.52	0.60	0.66	0.67
[voxels]	half sphere	0.23	0.27	0.36	0.37	0.55	0.55	0.48	0.40
II	polished	16.67	13.23	4.95	29.54	57.21	19.55	27.50	24.09
[μm]	periosteum	22.42	35.82	21.12	31.26	62.17	29.97	28.77	33.07

Remark 6.1. It should be noticed that the reference centroids of the second group were obtained indirectly by detecting the positions of the grid centre, which also contain deviations and are not 100% accurate. Unlike the reference centroids calculated analytically in the group I, the evaluation of group II can only give a rough impression about the accuracy of the algorithm.

6.2.3.2 Tracking with Multiple Landmarks

The experiments conducted in the previous section reveal that the single landmark detection is capable of a tracking with the accuracy on tens of micrometer scale. An even higher global tracking accuracy is expected while multiple landmarks are tracked using fiducial registration. In order to evaluate the whole tracking procedure, four landmark craters were ablated with the CO_2 laser on native bovine bone specimens, where the curved rough periosteum surface was retained, as shown in figure 6.7a. The landmarks were also 200 μm in diameter and 125 μm in depth. The geometric layout of the landmarks can be described as follows: if define the middle point of the landmark 2 and 4 as the origin and the line segment connecting them as the x-axis, where the direction $2 \rightarrow 4$ is defined as positive x-direction, then the landmarks 1 to 4 were located at $(0.25, -1.5), (-1.25, 0), (-0.25, 1)$ and $(1.25, 0)$ respectively.

A hexapod with the positioning accuracy of 2 μm and 10 μrad (figure 6.1b and table 6.1) was used as the external reference system. The sample was fixed to the platform of the hexapod and moved to pre-defined positions and orientations with high precision. OCT scans were acquired and the relative movement of the sample was tracked by the proposed tracking workflow (figure 6.7b). The resulting relative movements were compared with the actual movement performed by the hexapod and the tracking accuracy could be thus evaluated. Two groups of evaluations were conducted for translational and rotational accuracies respectively.

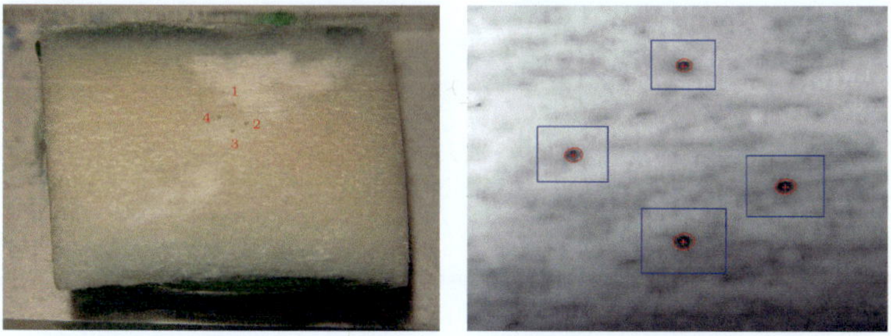

(a) (b)

Figure 6.7: (a) Tracking landmarks (marked with red numbers) ablated on native bovine bone specimen retaining original periosteum surface. (b) The detected landmark positions in OCT scan.

Translational Accuracy A cubic grid with the size of $2 \times 2 \times 2\,\mathrm{mm}^3$ containing 125 positions was chosen for evaluating the translational accuracy, defined as

$$\{(i/2, j/2, k/2)| -2 \leq i, j, k \leq 2 \wedge i, j, k \in \mathbb{Z}\}$$

The distance between neighbouring grid point is hence 0.5 mm. The sample was positioned to these grid points one by one, while its orientation was kept constant, yielding 124 test movements. A further coordinate system registration was performed to generate the reference vectors in the directions of i, j, k respectively. Taking the i-direction as example, two extra OCT scan were acquired at the positions $(-3/2, 0, 0)$ and $(3/2, 0, 0)$. Normalizing the relative movement between these two scans and set its length to 0.5 mm, the reference vector could be obtained.

For each test movement, the relative translations $\mathbf{t}$ calculated from the step 5 of the fiducial registration (section 6.2.2.3) were compared with the corresponding reference vectors. The mean absolute error between the results of the tracking and the reference vectors was $22.8 \pm 14.9\,\mu\mathrm{m}$ and the corresponding root mean square was $27.2\,\mu\mathrm{m}$. Figure 6.8 shows the distribution of the absolute tracking errors. It could further be determined that in 83.7% cases the tracking error was less than $40\,\mu\mathrm{m}$ while 96.8% were less than $50\,\mu\mathrm{m}$. The maximal error was $75.6\,\mu\mathrm{m}$.

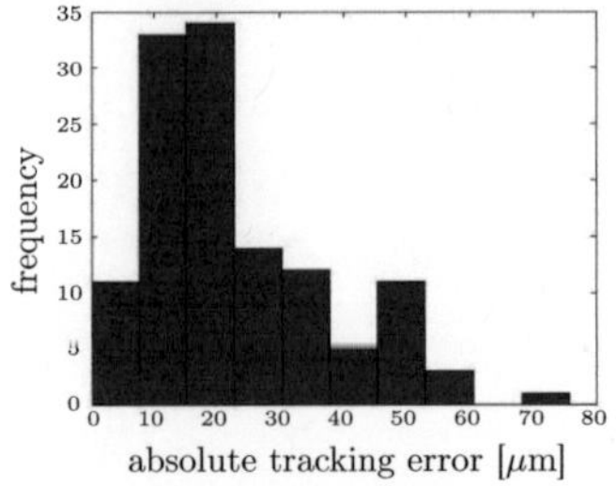

Figure 6.8: Distribution of absolute translational tracking errors.

Rotational Accuracy To evaluate the rotational accuracy, the sample was rotated about the X, Y and Z axes of the hexapod (see figure 6.1b) from $-12°$ to $12°$ respectively, where the sample orientation at $-12°$ is regarded as zero position. Knowing the rotation axis and the angle, it was trivial to generate a reference rotation matrix R_{ref} describing the actual rotation performed by the hexapod, which is compared with the rotation matrix R obtained from the step 4 of the fiducial registration by calculating $R_{\text{diff}} = R^t_{\text{ref}} \cdot R$, denoting the difference of the two rotations. The R_{diff} is then transformed to the quaternion expression in the form of $(\cos\theta/2, \mathbf{q}\sin\theta/2)$, where the unit vector $\mathbf{q} = (q_x, q_y, q_z)$ denotes the corresponding rotation axis while θ is the rotation angle. θ is exactly the rotational error in this case and the resulting absolute rotational errors are listed in table 6.3, where the mean absolute error was $0.21° \pm 0.20°$ and the root mean square was $0.28°$.

Table 6.3: Rotational accuracy (absolute error) of the proposed tracking mechanism using the four landmarks shown in figure 6.7, unit: °.

rotation axis	3°	6°	9°	12°	15°	18°	21°	24°
X	0.29	0.74	0.50	0.24	0.69	0.15	0.03	0.02
Y	0.18	0.07	0.46	0.06	0.07	0.20	0.03	0.19
Z	0.24	0.06	0.04	0.21	0.09	0.04	0.20	0.12

6.2.4 Discussion

The evaluations in section 6.2.3.2 evidence that the proposed tracking mechanism is able to achieve a tracking accuracy only about $25\,\mu\text{m}$, about ten times so accurate as the conventional tracking system. The desired global tracking accuracy of less than 50 μm between the target area and the laser working space (figure 6.3b) is successfully realised.

Compared to the conventional tracking systems, the shortcomings stated at the end of section 6.2.1 no more exist for the proposed tracking mechanism. Thanks to the high resolution of the OCT, a high tracking accuracy of each single landmark has been reached (section 6.2.3.1). The complicated transformation chain from the target area to the laser working space has been bypassed by the new tracking mechanism, so that the tracking error accumulation due to this long chain will no more occur. The layout of the landmark craters surrounding the cochleostomy (figure 6.4) guarantees that the target area is located quasi at the centroid of the fiducial. The magnification of the rotational error due to the large distance between the fiducial centroid and the target area can hence be avoided. Our direct tracking mechanism is therefore inherent to be more accurate than the conventional tracking systems which track the target indirectly.

On the other hand, the rotational accuracy depends on the span of each rigid body individually. The larger the span is, the higher will the rotational accuracy be. Applying the same experimental evaluation described in section 6.2.3.2 to the NDI Polaris optical tracking system, we determined that the rotational tracking accuracy of the rigid body shown in figure 6.3a is 0.12° (RMS). Due to the much smaller diagonal size of the fiducial used for the evaluation (figure 6.7, $<$3mm), the rotational tracking error of the new tracking conception is about double so large (RMS 0.28°). Nevertheless, it should be noticed that similar as the translational tracking accuracy, the global rotational accuracy of the conventional tracking systems also suffers from the indirect tracking using multiple trackers. Moreover, the NDI Aurora electromagnetic tracking system provides the accuracy of 0.2-0.3° (RMS) for each tracker according to the official specification of the manufacturer. It can therefore be concluded that the rotational tracking accuracy of the proposed mechanism has at least as good as the conventional systems.

While choosing the landmark layout, it should be aware that the distance between landmarks shall be as large as possible in order to increase the rotational accuracy. Contrarily, the concrete layout such as symmetry does not play a role, because the search regions ensure that the landmarks detected in different scans can be spontaneously matched.

Currently, the major drawback of the proposed tracking mechanism is that a 3D OCT scan of the target area costs about 2-3 seconds per volume while the detection of the landmarks costs an extra second on an Intel Dual-Core E5300@2.6GHz with 8GB RAM Linux platform. The communication between the tracking module and the OCT via hard disk brings additional overhead. As a result, the tracking is currently still a "pseudo" one and the challenge for the future work is to achieve a tracking rate that is comparable to the conventional tracking systems. A multi-megahertz OCT [WBK+10, KWA+12] and a GPU-based tracking algorithm may provide the potential solution for this problem.

It should also be aware that the proposed tracking mechanism was designed for relatively small movements on sub-millimetre scale. If the movement is so large that the landmarks exceed the "search regions" (figure 6.4b) in the succeeding OCT scan, the next tracking loop will fail. Nevertheless, the conventional tracking systems are mature for tracking larger movements on millimetre scale. In the case of tracking failure, the rough position of the target area can first be determined using conventional tracking systems as usual and immediately apply the new mechanism afterwards for a more accurate tracking result. The new tracking conception is therefore not a replacement of, but a supplementary to the conventional systems, which extends the lower limit of the global tracking accuracy down to tens of micrometers.

Remark 6.2. The distortion of the scanning optics (detail see section 6.3.1) with respect to the real world is currently not taken into account. Hence, the tracking accuracy measured in section 6.2.3.2 actually contains the errors caused by the distortion. These errors are always nearly constant within a small area. In other words, the start and stop position of a tiny relative movement on hundred micrometer scale are distorted almost in the same direction with the same magnitude, while the tracking mechanism measures the difference between both positions. The locally constant distortion has therefore limited influence on the tracking accuracy. Nonetheless, an even higher accuracy would be expected if this distortion could be precisely corrected in future work.

6.2.5 Motion Compensation

Being able to track the movement of the patient with high accuracy, the spontaneous question is: how to compensate the detected movement?

Actually, describing the position change of a same point in two different OCT scans, the equation (6.2) can be directly used for correcting the relative movement between the patient and the OCT-CO_2 optics, known as *motion compensation.*

Reviewing the ablation planning introduced algorithm 5.4, the resulting ablation pattern is returned in the form of $AP = \{(x_i, y_i, z_i; \tau_i)\}$, where (x_i, y_i, z_i) describes the desired position of the i-th pulse in the OCT scan of the planning. Knowing the R and $\mathbf{t}$ describing the relative movement, the correct pulse position can be then intuitively calculated according to equation (6.2) as

$$(x_i, y_i, z_i)^t_{\text{cur}} = R \cdot (x_i, y_i, z_i)^t_{\text{plan}} + \mathbf{t} \tag{6.3}$$

Instead of the planned ablation pattern, the new positions $(x_i, y_i, z_i)_{\text{cur}}$ will be passed to the CO_2 laser controller. Correspondingly, the control loop of the OCT guided laser-cochleostomy proposed in figure 3.10 is modified as the following, which takes the actual position of the patient also into account.

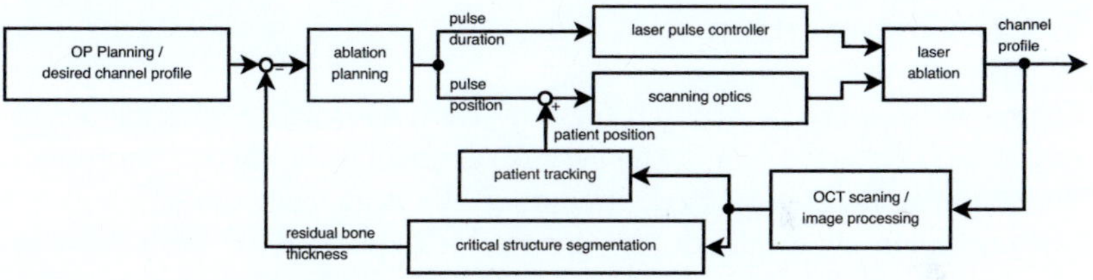

Figure 6.9: Control loop of the OCT guided laser-cochleostomy with patient tracking, where the patient movement is compensated using equation (6.3).

In addition, when a relative movement occurs, the position of the endosteum in the OCT scan will also be changed. Meanwhile, the concept of history compounding developed in section 5.2.2.2 requires the speckles from the same structure in different historical scans to be aligned together. Therefore, the equation (6.3) can also be used for aligning the speckles, where the $(x_i, y_i, z_i)^t_{\text{plan}}$ is simply replaced by the position of the involved voxels, yielding their positions in the new scan. The compounding can be then executed as usual.

6.3 Mapping between Scanning Optics

Until now, the control loop proposed in figure 6.9 is almost completed. The only missing step is to carry out the planned ablation pattern $AP = \{(x_i, y_i, z_i; \tau_i)\}$ by the CO_2 laser. While the pulse duration τ can be parsed by the laser pulse controller immediately, the pulse position (x, y, z) given in the OCT coordinate system can however not be directly executed by the CO_2 laser, whose scanning optics (see figure 2.8) has its own coordinate system that is completely different from that of the OCT. A mapping f between both coordinate systems is therefore vital for this final step. For a clear notation, the coordinates of a point given in the OCT and the CO_2 laser coordinate systems will be noted as (u, v, w) and (x, y, z) respectively in this section. The mapping f to be determined can be then written as:

$$\begin{aligned} f : \mathrm{OCT} &\rightarrow \mathrm{CO_2} \\ (u, v, w) &\mapsto (x, y, z) \end{aligned} \tag{6.4}$$

6.3.1 Observation

Before starting the determination of f, both coordinate systems are investigated more closely and the factors disturbing the correct coordinate transformation are analysed, including the scan field distortion, scan fields misalignment and trapezoidal working space of the both systems.

Scan Field Distortion As already introduced, both OCT and CO_2 laser systems are equipped with scanning optics to deflect the beam on a two dimensional scan field. Except the fan distortion in the axial direction along the laser beam[4] which was handled in section 5.1.2, the scanning mechanism also causes distortions in the other two directions. Figure 6.10a illustrates the distorted coordinate system of a scanner without focusing lens installed. Assuming that the incoming laser beam is perfectly adjusted and incident exactly onto the rotation axes of both mirrors and the laser beam hits the point A on the image field perpendicularly when both mirrors are at zero position.

[4] Actually, the scanning optics of CO_2 laser also leads to such a distortion. Nonetheless, the laser ablation is independent on the optical path length as long as the target surface is located within the working space of the laser (see figure 2.8). Therefore, there is no need to correct the fan-distortion for the CO_2 laser system.

When the x-mirror scans between zero position and some particular angle θ_x, the trace of the laser spot will form the line segment AB on the image field. Further scanning the y-mirror between zero and θ_y, the line segment AB will be translated between AB and CD on the image field. It can be immediately derived that the length of AB increases non-linearly with the θ_y, which results hence in a pillow-shaped distortion of the scan field shown in the illustration. In practice, it is often difficult to ensure the incoming beam to be incident exactly onto the axes of the mirrors, resulting in an extra trapezium-shaped distortion and makes the scan field asymmetric.

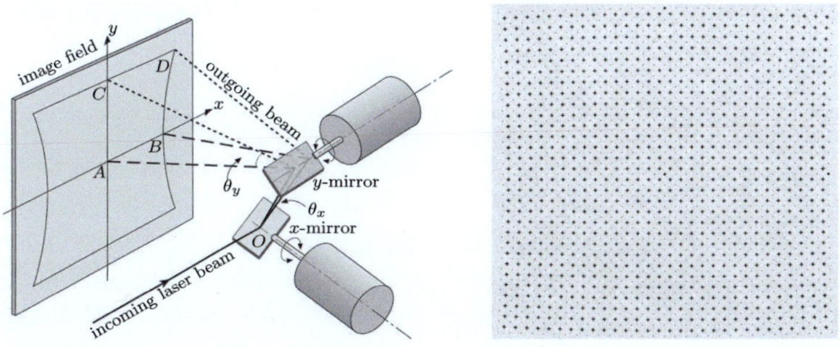

(a) (b)

Figure 6.10: (a) Field distortion of a double galvanometric scanning system without focusing lens [SCA06]. (b) A rectangular grid pattern ablated by the CO_2 laser with uncalibrated scanning optics on a piece of paper, which shows a pillow-barrel-shaped distortion.

In addition, both OCT and CO_2 laser scanners are equipped with focusing lens to achieve a tiny laser spot. Such a lens causes a further distortion which was already described in figure 5.6: a scanning mirror before the focal point results in a shrinking trend of the outgoing beam, intensifying the pillow-shaped distortion; a post-focal point mirror leads to a dilation trend, causing a barrel-shaped distortion. Consequently, the lens will bring additional distortion to the already distorted scan field shown in figure 6.10a. The final shape of the scan field depends on the combined action of the scanning mirrors and focusing lens. Figure 6.10b shows the distorted scan field of the CO_2 laser as an example, where a rectangular grid was ablated on a flat paper, which shows however a mixed pillow-barrel-shaped distortion. The scan field of the OCT has an analogous distortion.

Scan Fields Misalignment In addition to the distortions, the potential misalignment of the both scan fields makes the situation more complicated. Figure 6.11a illustrates the spatial relationship between the both coordinate systems of the coaxial setup (figure 6.1). Due to the unavoidable inaccuracy while attaching the OCT to the CO_2 laser, both origins could be misaligned and the whole CO_2 laser coordinate system could be slightly rotated against that of the OCT.

In addition to the in plane misalignment, the CO_2 laser optics is even very likely to be a little bit inclined with respect to the OCT, so that the red optical path (CO_2 laser) is not necessarily parallel to the purple optical path (OCT) in the illustration. As a result, both focal planes as well as the z- and w-axis are probably not parallel to each other.

Trapezoidal Working Spaces A further difficulty is that the laser beam is perpendicular to the focal plane if and only if the mirrors are at zero position, which is inclined at any other mirror positions with $\theta_x \neq 0$ or $\theta_y \neq 0$. As a result, the working space (refer to figure 2.8) of the both scanning optics are trapezium-shaped rather than rectangular, as illustrated in figure 6.11b. The size of the scan fields is therefore changing along the optical axes. In other words, while being projected onto the focal plane, two points (x, y, z_1) and (x, y, z_2) are not overlapped for the same mirror position (x, y) in the CO_2 laser coordinate system, if $z_1 \neq z_2$. The OCT has the same problem.

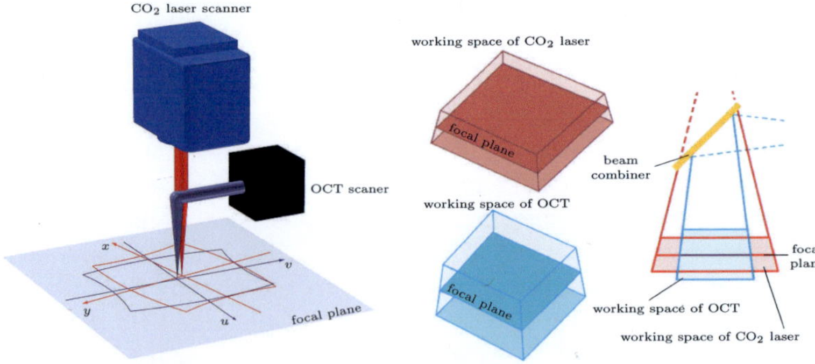

(a) (b)

Figure 6.11: Illustrations of (a) scan fields misalignment due to unavoidable inaccuracy while attaching the OCT to the CO_2 laser; (b) trapezoidal working spaces of both scanning optics.

6.3.2 Determination of the Mapping

6.3.2.1 Analysis

While determining the mapping between both coordinate systems, all the factors described above have to be taken into account. Having been widely used since decades, correction of the scan field distortion of a single scanning optics is already a mature technology. However, a calibration and registration technology for a double scanners system in our case does not exist yet. Nevertheless, an intuitive three-steps approach can be easily conceived as:

i. Choose an appropriate existing distortion correction technique and correct the field distortion of the OCT and CO_2 laser separately.

ii. Coordinate system registration between the corrected scan fields, so that the scan fields misalignment can be easily compensated.

iii. Determine the zoom factor along the optical axis.

The key step of this chain is the correction of the field distortion. In the following, the existing techniques will be shortly reviewed.

Correction of Scan Field Distortion: A Short Review Wu [Wu87] created a mathematical model describing the double galvanometric scanning system with a focusing lens. Based on this model, the field distortion can be analytically deduced and hence corrected correspondingly. This model requires the incoming beam to be precisely incident onto the rotation axes of the mirrors, which is however difficult to be achieved in practice. The modelling of such a system with an improperly incident beam is very complicated, so that the most techniques nowadays are based on measuring the distorted field directly.

The simplest but most common approach is to describe the distorted scan field by fitting or interpolating the grid points in the distorted scan field (for example the figure 6.10b) with a piecewise bi-quadratic or bi-cubic polynomial [CC07, HFI+08, CCH09], while Xie et al. [XHD+05] only utilized nine points (the four corners, centre points of the four edges and the origin) for the interpolation.

For commercial use, the control software InScript (ARGES GmbH, Germany) of our CO_2 laser system provides another approach. The technique chooses some particular feature points on the distorted scan field.

By measuring the distance between them, a correction pattern dual to the distorted scan field can be generated accordingly (6.12a).

These approaches have however a limitation that the correction is two dimensional and only valid for the single plane, in which the calibration was performed. In practice, the correction is often performed on the focal plane and considered to be still valid within some tolerance range above and below it if neglecting the error induced by the distance to the focal plane. For our case, the correction errors of the two scanning optics will be accumulated, which could also further affect the succeeding coordinate system registration and zoom factor determination. Therefore, a pure three-dimensional correction method is preferred.

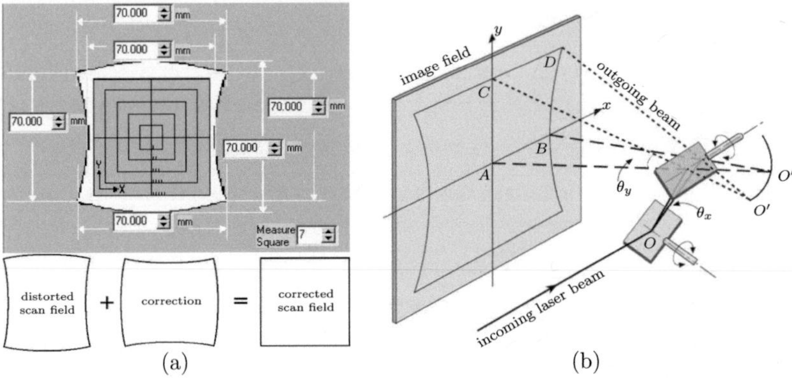

Figure 6.12: (a) Correction method provided by InScript software (ARGES GmbH, Germany). The correction pattern is generated according to the distances measured between particular feature points on the distorted scan field [ARG08]. (b) For a double galvanometric scanning system, the trace of projection centres is not a fixed point but forms an arc $O'O''$, whose radius is exactly the distance between the two mirrors, modified from figure 6.10a [SCA06].

For the three-dimensional case, Cui et al. [CZWX09] tried to adapt a pinhole camera model to describe the scanning optics and then apply the famous camera calibration technique of Zhang [Zha00]. However, this approach is theoretically incorrect, because the camera model assumes that there exists an optical centre, through which all projection lines must pass. Unfortunately, such a point does not exist in the double galvanometric scanning system, as illustrated in figure 6.12b. It can be derived that the trace of the intersection points of the outgoing beams is an arc due to the rotation of the y-mirror. The camera model is therefore not capable of describing the scanning optics. As a result, the calibration error of the approach of Cui et al. was one order of magnitude higher than the other methods, which is on millimetre scale for a $150 \times 150\,\text{mm}^2$ scan field while the above polynomial interpolation based approaches had an accuracy of about 100-150 μm and 10-30 μm for scan fields with the size of $300 \times 300\,\text{mm}^2$ and $30 \times 30\,\text{mm}^2$ respectively [XHD+05, CC07].

Recently, Manakov et al. [MSI11] tried to correct the distortion in 3D by means of creating mathematical model for the scanning system. The model takes the above mentioned improperly incident beam also into account. However, the authors modelled only the double galvanometric scanning system without focusing lens. A mathematical modelling of the scanning optics with lens installed like our case still remains unsolved.

Therefore, the only available choice is the single plane correction methods, which is however not accurate enough for our three-dimensional double scanner case. The combined influences of the inaccuracy with the succeeding steps is also unpredictable. In addition, while the distorted scan field of the CO_2 laser can be easily obtained by ablating a grid on a paper or other flat material surface, it is difficult to record the scan field of the OCT. A high resolution infrared camera or infrared-sensitive film might be a solution, which however significantly increases the complexity and cost of the procedure. In conclusion, the above conceived three-steps approach based on existing mature techniques is unfortunately not practical.

6.3.2.2 Tri-Cubic B-Spline Fitting based Registration

Considering the disadvantage of the three-steps approach, a pure three-dimensional registration covering all factors introduced in section 6.3.1 with minimal possible steps is desired. It was noticed that, if the CO_2 laser ablates a crater at the position (x, y, z), the corresponding coordinate (u, v, w) of the crater centroid in the OCT coordinate system can be directly detected by algorithm 6.1, yielding a point pair from both coordinate systems.

This provides immediately another simple thread for finding the mapping f within a single step. The main idea is to extend the polynomial fitting based single plane correction method to the third dimension: first, a point cloud filling the whole working space will be ablated by the CO_2 laser. With the help of the landmark detection algorithm, the corresponding point cloud in the OCT coordinate system can be easily obtained. By means of a three dimensional polynomial fitting of these points pairs, the mapping f can be determined without any intermediate steps. A high accuracy can be hence expected.

Generation of Point Cloud Due to the size limit of the beam combiner, the common part of the both working spaces is about $10 \times 10 \times 3\,\mathrm{mm}^3$ (L×W×H). Considering the slightly misaligned origins and coordinate axes, a two-dimensional registration grid with the size of $14 \times 14\,\mathrm{mm}^2$ was defined within the CO_2 laser coordinate system as

$$\{(x, y) | -7 \leq x, y \leq 7\} \cup \{(x + 0.5, y + 0.5) | -7 \leq x, y \leq 6\} \quad (6.5)$$

where $x, y \in \mathbb{Z}$, as shown in figure 6.13a. The size of the crater at the origin is doubled, so that it can be distinguished from other points.

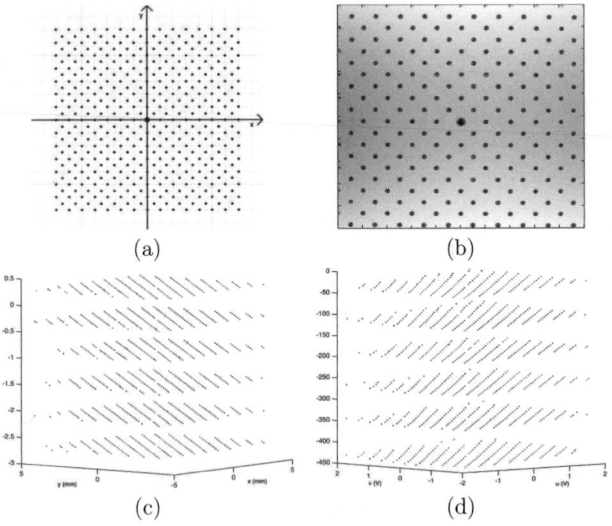

Figure 6.13: (a) Two-dimensional registration grid defined in the CO_2 coordinate system and (b) the corresponding points detect in the OCT coordinate system. (c-d) The corresponding point pairs filling the whole common working space in (c) the CO_2 laser and (d) the OCT coordinate systems. The blue points are the original point pairs and the red ones are calculated by the mappings f and f^{-1} obtained from the tri-cubic B-spline fitting for a qualitative examination.

Starting from the top of the common working space, a flat acrylic plate was used as target surface and the grid defined by equation (6.5) was ablated by the CO_2 laser on it. An OCT scan of the acrylic plate was acquired and the algorithm 6.1 was applied to determine the corresponding points, as shown in figure 6.13b. Moreover, instead of using the centroid position returned by the algorithm, each detected grid point (u, v, w) was projected onto the acrylic plate surface in the OCT scan. It could hence be ensured that the obtained w coordinates were exactly corresponding to the surface position z in the CO_2 laser coordinate system.

With the help of the hexapod, the acrylic plate was precisely translated along the z-axis downwards to the next predefined position. Repeating the above ablation-detection-translation procedure until the complete common working space was covered, the point cloud for the fitting could be obtained. Considering the common working space with the height of 3 mm, six equidistant z-positions with the step length of 0.6 mm were chosen. The resulting point clouds in the CO_2 laser and the OCT coordinate systems are plotted in figure 6.13c-d with blue points.

Tri-Cubic B-Spline Fitting Considering that the most mature technologies have described the field distortion on a single plane with piecewise bi-quadratic or bi-cubic polynomials, while the misalignment between the coordinate systems is an affine map and the field zoom along the optical axes is linear, it is reasonable to assume that the three-dimensional mapping between the OCT and the CO_2 laser coordinate systems can also be approximated by piecewise tri-cubic polynomials. The tri-cubic B-spline fitting technique is hence chosen to solve the approximation problem due to its excellent smoothness, affine invariance, flexibility and simplicity.

Suppose there exist totally m point pairs $(\mathbf{p}_i, \mathbf{q}_i)$ with $\mathbf{p}_i = (u_i, v_i, w_i)$ and $\mathbf{q}_i = (x_i, y_i, z_i)$ in the point cloud. The tri-cubic B-spline fitting problem can be simply established by solving the following linear system:

$$\mathbf{N}(u, v, w)\mathbf{C} = \mathbf{Q}$$

where

$$\mathbf{N}(u, v, w) = \begin{bmatrix} N_0^3(u_0)N_0^3(v_0)N_0^3(w_0) & \cdots & N_j^3(u_0)N_k^3(v_0)N_l^3(w_0) \\ \vdots & & \vdots \\ N_0^3(u_m)N_0^3(v_m)N_0^3(w_m) & \cdots & N_j^3(u_m)N_k^3(v_m)N_l^3(w_m) \end{bmatrix}$$

and $\mathbf{C} = [\mathbf{c}_{000}^t, \cdots, \mathbf{c}_{jkl}^t]^t$, $\mathbf{Q} = [\mathbf{q}_0^t, \cdots, \mathbf{q}_m^t]^t$ respectively. $\mathbf{C}$ is the control polygon of the tri-cubic B-spline volume and $N_i^n(u)$ denotes the n degree B-spline recursive formula of the i-th control point (definition and more details refer to [PBP02]).

Solving this over determined system by applying least squares fitting:

$$\mathbf{C} = (\mathbf{N}^t\mathbf{N})^{-1}\mathbf{N}^t\mathbf{Q} \tag{6.6}$$

the control polygon describing the three-dimensional mapping f from the OCT coordinate system to the CO_2 laser coordinate system can be obtained, yielding the analytical expression of the equation (6.4):

$$f(u, v, w) = \left[\ N_0^3(u)N_0^3(v)N_0^3(w) \quad \cdots \quad N_j^3(u)N_k^3(v)N_l^3(w)\ \right] \mathbf{C}$$

which is calculated by applying the *de Boor* algorithm (refer to [PBP02]) in practice. When necessary, the inverse function f^{-1} from the CO_2 laser system back to the OCT system can also be simply obtained by swapping the $\mathbf{p}$ and $\mathbf{q}$ in the above equation system, yielding $\mathbf{N}(x, y, z)\mathbf{C} = \mathbf{P}$ and solve it accordingly.

Evaluation For a preliminary qualitative examination, the obtained f and f^{-1} were applied to the original point cloud $\{\mathbf{p}_i\}$ and $\{\mathbf{q}_i\}$ respectively. The resulting $f(u_i, v_i, w_i)$ and $f^{-1}(x_i, y_i, z_i)$ with $i = 1, \cdots, m$ are plotted into figure 6.13c-d with red dots. It can be observed that the calculated points match the original ones very well in both cases.

For a quantitative evaluation, a mapping error between a point pair $\mathbf{p} = (u, v, w)$ and $\mathbf{q} = (x, y, z)$ is defined as

$$\epsilon(\mathbf{p}, \mathbf{q}) = |(x, y, z) - f(u, v, w)| \tag{6.7}$$

where $|\cdot|$ denotes the vector length. Applying equation (6.7) to all m point pairs, a mean mapping error of 12.1 μm was obtained.

Noticing that these m point pairs had already been used for the determination of f, the mapping error between them can be actually considered as a measure for the quality of the fitting by applying the equation (6.6). For a more strict evaluation, a new evaluation grid was defined as:

$$\begin{aligned} &\{(x, y + 0.5)| - 7 \leq x \leq 7, -7 \leq y \leq 6\} \\ \cup &\{(x + 0.5, y)| - 7 \leq x \leq 6, -7 \leq y \leq 7\} \end{aligned}$$

which is the set of the middle points in every rhombus of the registration grid (figure 6.13a) defined by equation (6.5). Meanwhile, the five middle points between the six positions used for the registration were chosen as evaluation positions. The acrylic plate was translated to these positions and the evaluation pattern defined above was ablated on it. The same ablation-detection-translation procedure as the registration was performed at the evaluation positions. A second evaluation point cloud containing the points with the maximal distances to the m registration points was thus generated.

Qualitative examination of the evaluation point cloud yielded similar results as figure 6.13c-d. The mean mapping error among the evaluation points was $29.3\,\mu$m, which is although larger than that among the registration points but still accurate enough. The mean mapping error of all registration and evaluation point pairs was $19.6\,\mu$m.

6.3.3 Discussion

Although no strict mathematical proof has been made, the result of the evaluation reveals that approximating the mapping f between the OCT and the CO_2 laser coordinate systems with tri-cubic B-splines is accurate enough. On the other hand, it should be noticed that while evaluating the mapping accuracy according to equation (6.7), the (u, v, w) were detected by applying algorithm 6.1 in the acquired OCT scans. Consequently, the landmark detection error of the algorithm is also included in the mapping errors obtained above. Therefore, these results give not only a measure about the accuracy of the mapping f alone, but can actually be regarded as the global error of the complete patient tracking-coordinate mapping procedure to some extent. Of course, further experiments specifically designed for this evaluation are required for a more persuasive conclusion.

In addition to the factors stated in section 6.3.1, the proposed method also covers the fan-distortion of the OCT volume (refer to section 5.1.2). In order to prove this point, the above registration and evaluation were actually conducted without correcting the fan-distortion, which can be perceived in figure 6.13b and d, where the extracted surface and point cloud are slightly curved. As a result, the accuracy of the fan-distortion correction will not directly affect the final precision of the ablation.

6.4 Experimental Evaluation

Up to now, all issues in the control loop proposed in figure 6.9 have been solved and the desired closed-loop control of the laser ablation is thereby successfully established. The complete workflow was experimentally evaluated by conducting the worldwide first OCT guided laser-cochleostomy on porcine cochleae isolated from cadavers.

Standard Bone Sheet Before performing the cochleostomy on real cochleae, the whole workflow was first tested on artificial specimens with simple structures already known, so that potential system bugs can be found and fixed more easily. Fresh bovine bone sheets with the size of circa $30 \times 30 \times 1\,\mathrm{mm}^3$ were therefore manually polished and then fixed on an acrylic plate (figure 6.14a). The interface between the bone sheet and acrylic plate was regarded as the critical structure, so that the specimen has a simple but defined structure for the preliminary experiment.

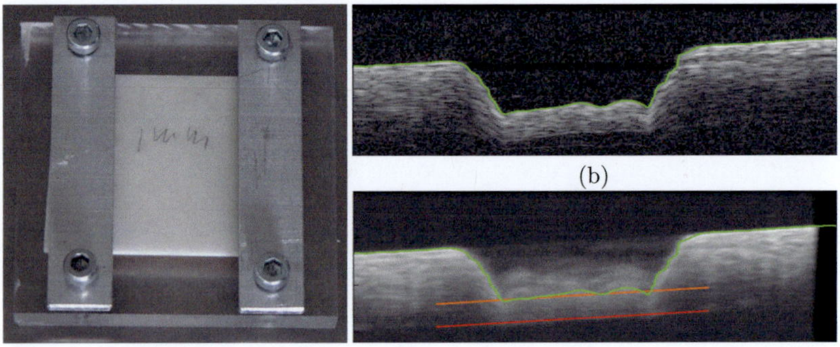

(a) (b) (c)

Figure 6.14: Qualitative trial of the workflow on a standard bone sheet: (a) the specimen; (b) the refractive index compensated B-scan passing through the center of the dummy insertion channel after the termination of the ablation, the green curve is the sample surface; (c) the same frame showing the enhanced B-scan using history compounding (section 5.2.2.2) and the segmented critical structure (red) as well as the stop surface (orange). The propagation of the channel bottom has been captured by history compounding. The black column on the right margin is the trace of the specimen movement during the ablation process.

Dummy cochleostomy were ablated on the bone sheet. Before starting the ablation, four landmark craters surrounding the intended channel position were ablated for patient tracking (example see figure 6.17). During the succeeding ablation, water spray was manually applied onto the ablation area using syringe to avoid laser ablation induced thermal injury (refer to section 2.2.2). Meanwhile, the water spray also prevented tissue dehydration that can severely disturb the OCT imaging of the critical structure. Slight random movements of the specimen was generated by touching the surrounding tissue with the syringe needle.

The control loop of the laser ablation was then started. Noticing that two different criteria equation (5.19) and (5.20) were defined for algorithm 5.4 which determines the next pulse positions. Experiments on standard bone sheets revealed that the strategy based on equation (5.20) can achieve better results. While an undesired V-shaped valley has been formed (example see figure 5.31a), equation (5.19) often guides the laser to be shot into the valley, because the accumulative thickness reaches the maximal at the tip of the "V" due to the large bone thickness on the wall of the valley. This pulse will naturally make the situation worth.

On the contrary, equation (5.20) plans two pulses on both sides of the valley opening in such a case, so that the valley depth will be reduced, resulting in a smoother channel bottom. Figure 6.14b-c shows the effect of applying the algorithm 5.4 using the equation (5.20). Considering the gaussian-shaped craters ablated by each single laser pulse (figure 5.29a-b), the smoothness of the resulting channel bottom is already very well. In the following, all ablation are planned using criterion equation (5.20).

Fresh Porcine Cochlea Having verified the workflow with the simple standard bone sheet, the developed control loop is finally ready to perform the cochleostomy. Three cochleostomies were performed. No preoperative planning was made and the cochleae were manually positioned and oriented in the laser working space. The position of the bone-endosteum-perilymph boundary was unknown while starting the ablation process. Therefore, the achieved accuracy was completely dependent on the proposed workflow. Figure 6.15 shows the changing channel shape during one of the cochleostomies.

At the early stage of the ablation (sub-figure a-c), the bone-endosteum-perilymph boundary was still barely visible due to the relatively thick overlying bone layer. During this phase, the ablation was planned according to a virtual critical structure located at infinity and parallel to the original bone surface (pre-segmentation phase, refer to algorithm

5.4 and relevant texts), resulting in a channel bottom approximately parallel to it. With the increasing channel depth, the critical structure became gradually visible (sub-figure d). After applying the image quality enhancement and critical structure segmentation (sections 5.2 and 5.3), the ablation could be planned according to the bone thickness distribution measured online. As a result, the channel bottom began to incline clockwise and its shape converged to that of the endosteal layer step by step as expected (sub-figured d-i).

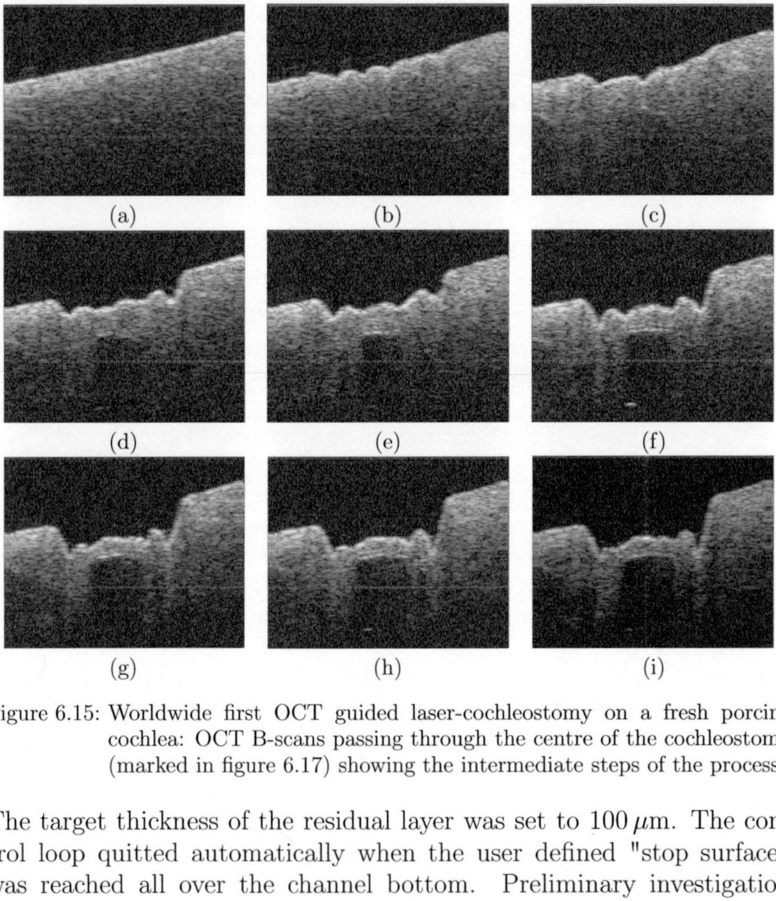

Figure 6.15: Worldwide first OCT guided laser-cochleostomy on a fresh porcine cochlea: OCT B-scans passing through the centre of the cochleostomy (marked in figure 6.17) showing the intermediate steps of the process.

The target thickness of the residual layer was set to 100 μm. The control loop quitted automatically when the user defined "stop surface" was reached all over the channel bottom. Preliminary investigation in postoperative OCT scans indicates that the shape of the resulting cochleostomy macroscopically matches the curvature of the cochlear endosteum (figure 6.16a-c).

Instead of only evaluating the ablation accuracy at a single point, a more strict evaluation comparing the whole channel bottom with the "stop surface" was performed (Figure 9d). According to the measurement in the postoperative OCT scan, the mean absolute errors between the resulting channel bottom and the three-dimensional "stop surface" were 16.43±14.90, 19.62±17.67 and 21.01±21.39 μm for the three cochleostomies respectively. The corresponding maximal errors where the channel bottom penetrated the "stop surface" were 45.54 μm, 38.36 μm and 46.73 μm. An evaluation of the accuracy based on histological studies is still to be made.

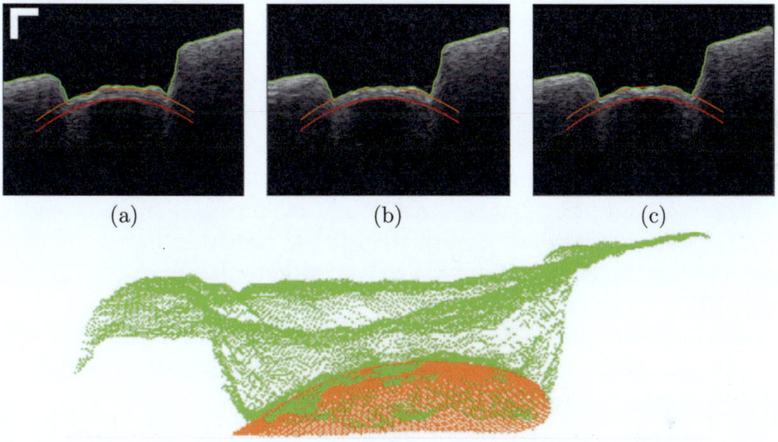

(a) (b) (c) (d)

Figure 6.16: (a-c) Example OCT B-scans acquired near the center of a resulting cochleostomy, showing the final shape of the ablated cochleostomy, bar=250 μm. (d) Comparison between the resulting channel bottom (green) and the three-dimensional "stop surface" (orange).

The top view of the resulting cochleostomy under the OCT is shown in figure 6.17a and further microscopic inspection was performed to investigate the laser ablation induced thermal injury (figure 6.17b). It can be observed that the bottom of the cochleostomy is very clean and no obvious carbonisation can be discovered.

In conclusion, the developed OCT guided laser-cochleostomy system has successfully achieved an ablation accuracy on tens of micrometer scale without bringing severe thermal injury to the surrounding tissues.

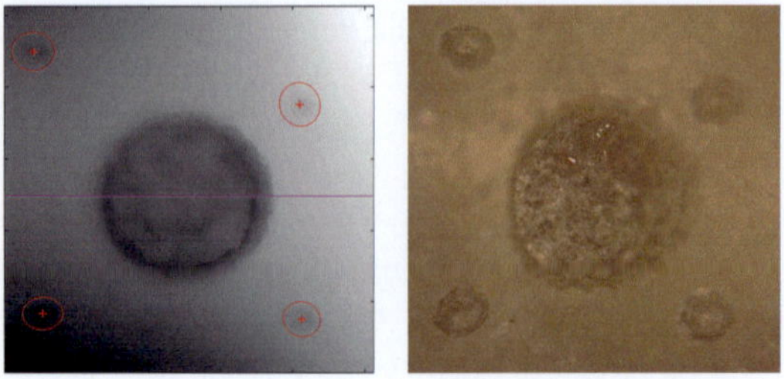

(a) (b)

Figure 6.17: The resulting cochleostomy and the landmark craters (a) in the OCT and (b) under microscope, where the violet line denotes the position of the B-scans shown in figure 6.15.

Discussion The preliminary result of the experimental evaluation reveals that under the monitoring of the OCT, the laser ablation can be directly guided according to the residual bone thickness above the bone-endosteum-perilymph boundary measured online. In contrast to the control conceptions using other sensor technologies (refer to section 2.3.2), a foresighted detection of the critical structure before its exposure has been realised. Compared to the workgroups who have also been using OCT to guide the laser ablation [FSK+12, DKG+13, LWFY12], our approach does not only rely on measuring the bone surface but takes the full advantage of the tomographic information provided by the high resolution imaging system.

A unique feature of our system is that the laser control module does not only control the laser on and laser off, but also optimises pulse positions and pulse durations according to the residual bone thickness distribution. To our knowledge, a uniform convergence of the resulting channel bottom to the shape of the critical structure has been demonstrated for the first time. Reviewing the control loop, it can also be noticed that the workflow is independent on the type of the integrated ablating laser. The CO_2 laser in the setup (figure 6.1a) can be replaced by other kind of surgical lasers such as the commonly used Er:YAG laser.

On the other hand, our system is still an experimental setup and we have a long way to go before bringing it into real operation room. It can be observed that the resulting cochleostomy is not perfect and there exist in all three cochleostomies some positions where the channel bottom has penetrated the "stop surface" (figure 6.16), indicating that a 100% protection of the endosteum has not been guaranteed yet.

Meanwhile, the critical structure segmentation is not fully automatic yet. Due to the limited imaging depth of OCT, the critical structure is always invisible at the beginning (figure 6.15a) or only a few pixels can be seen in the middle part (figure 6.15b-c). The segmentation is impossible in the first case and often returns a wrong result in the later one. A manual correctness check of segmentation result is still mandatory. Further improvement of the ablation strategy and a more intelligent segmentation algorithm are therefore necessary.

Time consumption is another critical issue in the current system implementation. The OCT imaging, processing and the CO_2 laser control are done by three independent software packages and a manual data transfer between them is required. This has led to unnecessary overhead and allows human error to happen. Depending on the initial conditions including bone thickness and shape of the underlying endosteal layer, the OCT guided laser cochleostomy may cost up to more than one hour. Due to the manual data transfer, a real time tracking of the patient movements using the proposed tracking mechanism is impossible in the current state, either. Further works should still be done on speeding up the process by unifying the software packages and implementing GPU-based algorithms. Extensive systematic evaluations regarding the reliability, robustness and repeatability of the system under different conditions are also essential.

6.5 Summary

In this chapter, the integration of the OCT and the CO_2 laser system is successfully realised. Having discovered that the accuracy of conventional marker based optical tracking systems does not match the high accuracy of the OCT guided laser ablation system, an innovative concept of using the OCT itself as an optical tracking system is proposed. A mean absolute tracking error of about $25\,\mu m$ was achieved, which is more than ten times so accurate as the conventional systems. A precise three-dimensional mapping with a global mean absolute error of $19.6\,\mu m$ between both scanning optics has been determined, enabling a precise execution of the ablation pattern planned in the OCT system by the CO_2 laser. The control loop of the laser ablation is hence completed and the system was experimentally evaluated. The result of the preliminary experiment on fresh porcine cochleae evidences that a precise approaching of the critical structure with an accuracy on tens of micrometer scale has been achieved. The desired closed-loop control of the laser-cochleostomy under the monitoring of the OCT is thereby successfully established.

CHAPTER 7

Summary and Outlook

Within the scope of this doctoral thesis, an optical coherence tomography guided laser-cochleostomy system is proposed and successfully developed. Under the monitoring of the OCT, the position of the fragile cochlear endosteum can be detected several hundred micrometres in advance, so that the laser ablation can foresightedly approach the shape of the critical structure (see figure 6.15a) and duly terminate as soon as the pre-defined thickness of the tissue layer to be preserved is reached (see figure 6.15b-c). A closed-loop control of the endosteum preserving laser-cochleostomy (figure 7.1) with an accuracy on tens of micrometre scale is established.

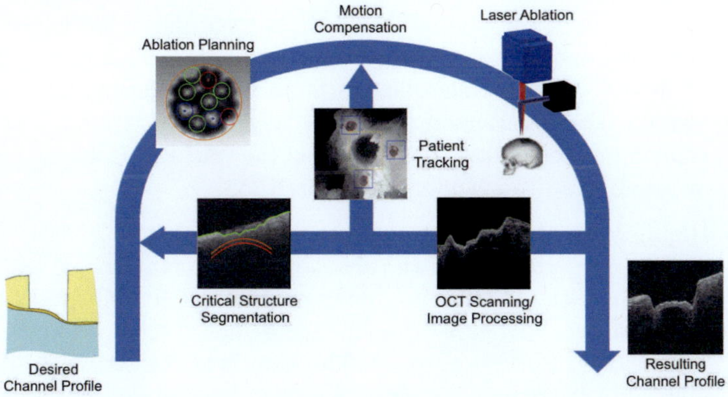

Figure 7.1: Control loop of OCT guided endosteum preserving laser-cochleostomy.

7.1 Summary

In summary, the following scientific highlights are achieved in this work:

- Residual bone thickness based control:
  Compared to other control concepts stated in section 2.3.2, our control loop is the only one that can plan the laser ablation foresightedly based on the online measured residual bone thickness above the critical structure. The other approaches can either detect the tissue boundary only after the first pulse applied to the underlying soft tissue (laser ablation induced emissions based approaches), or control the ablation indirectly by monitoring the ablation depth (ultrasound, confocal microscopy).

- Refractive index measurement using OCT:
  Without knowing the refractive index of the bony shell of the cochlea, OCT itself is used for measuring this important parameter, which is also capable to determine the refractive index for each patient individually during the operation (refer to section 5.1.3.4).

- History compounding:
  The speckle noises in OCT images significantly compromise the ability of OCT to resolve the critical structures. The simple but effective history compounding technique can considerably improve the image quality and make the succeeding segmentation much easier (refer to section 5.2.2.2).

- OCT as optical tracking system:
  Working with the accuracy on tens of micrometre scale, the conventional marker based optical tracking system with the accuracy of several hundred micrometres is no more sufficient for our situation. The OCT itself is innovatively used as a precise optical tracking system, which has improved the tracking accuracy for one order of magnitude (refer to section 6.2).

- Highly accurate mapping between scanning optics:
  The precise execution of the ablation pattern requires an accurate three-dimensional mapping between the OCT and the laser ablation system. A tri-cubic B-spline fitting based calibration method is developed for this purpose. The scan field distortion, misalignment and trapezoidal working space of both scanning optics are calibrated in a single step (refer to section 6.3).

Compared to the accuracy of <0.5 mm achieved by other researchers [FSK+12, FKS+12, DKG+13] who also attempted to guide the laser bone ablation with OCT, the OCT guided laser-cochleostomy system developed in this work is one order of magnitude more accurate. The main drawback of the system proposed by these researchers is, the control was only based on the reconstructed bone surface profile while the valuable tomographic information about the micro-structures beneath the bone surface delivered by OCT was abandoned. Meanwhile, the authors had not taken the complicated workspace distortions of both laser systems into account and simply described the mapping between the two coordinate systems with a rigid transformation, which further reduced the accuracy of their approach.

In conclusion, the highly accurate OCT guided laser-cochleostomy system developed in this thesis provides an "eye" to the laser bone ablation, which brings more safety and less trauma to the patient and relieves the stress on the surgeon during the operation as well.

7.2 Outlook

7.2.1 Adaptation to Other Micro-Surgeries

Being able to perform the endosteum preserving laser-cochleostomy under the guidance of an OCT, the next question raised is: *Would it be possible to adapt this technique to other kinds of micro-surgeries?*

After reviewing each single step developed in chapter 5 and chapter 6, it can be concluded that most of the steps are independent from the type of micro-surgery and can be applied to other cases directly except the detection of cochlear endosteum (section 5.3) and ablation planning (section 5.4). The endosteum detection is based on the fact that the structure has a dark-bright-dark appearance in the enhanced OCT images. The appearance of other critical structures in OCT images might probably be different. Meanwhile, specialized OCT are often used for imaging of some specific tissues, such as Doppler-OCT for blood flow measurement [IKY+97, ZFSS00, LIS+09], polarization diversity OCT for nerve fibers [Sch99, ZJNC04, MYY09a] etc. Therefore, while adapting the control loop to a new case, a detailed analysis of the structure property is mandatory in order to design an appropriate workflow.

Meanwhile, the ablation planning developed in section 5.4 is designed to create a cylindrical insertion channel. For incision with other geometries, a new ablation strategy is necessary.

7.2.2 Robot Assisted OCT Scanning

Similar to the robot assisted laser osteotomy system introduced in section 2.3.1, a robot[1] would also considerably improve the performance of the OCT guided laser ablation in the following aspects:

- Extended working space:
  A significant shortcoming of the OCT is, its scan field is very limited. Most commercial models provide only 10×10 to $20 \times 20\,\text{mm}^2$ scanning area, which makes the imaging of large objects difficult. With the help of a robot, the working space of an OCT can be almost "unlimitedly" extended. A larger area can be covered by repositioning the OCT and concatenating the acquired scans.
- Spatial compounding for speckle noise reduction:
  As already proposed in figure 5.20, the robot permits a flexible observation of an object from arbitrary incident angles, enabling the speckle noise reduction by spatial compounding without resolution trade-off (details refer to relevant texts of figure 5.20).
- Working distance compensation:
  As stated, the tissue surface to be processed has to be located near the focal plane within the Rayleigh range (refer to section 2.2.1 and figure 2.8) of both lasers. However, while ablating a deep structure, the bottom of the incision might exceed the lower boundary of the working spaces. Such a case can be easily recognized in OCT scans and then compensated by the robot.

7.2.3 OCT-Acoustics Based Hybrid Control

Although the OCT works excellently for guiding the laser-cochleostomy, the system is however not capable of monitoring narrow but deep incisions like the examples shown in figure 7.2a. It can be observed that

[1] Compared with serial kinematics, more stable and more accurate parallel kinematics (hexapod) are more capable for our case.

the width at the incision bottom is only about 20-30 μm, corresponding to 1-3 pixels with typical scanning density (number of A-scans per millimetre), which are insufficient for a segmentation (figure 7.2b).

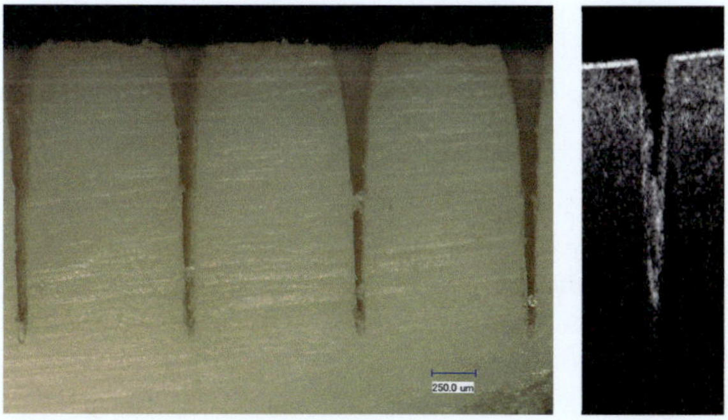

(a) (b)

Figure 7.2: (a) Cross section view of laser ablated narrow but deep incisions under microscope, bar=250 μm; (b) OCT scan of such an incision.

In such a case, a foresighted detection of the underlying soft tissue is no more possible. As a result, the ablation control has to rely on the ablation depth measured from the bone surface profile. As analysed in section 2.3.2, the indirect ablation control based on the online measured ablation depth would probably not be accurate enough. This deduction is also evidenced by the relatively low accuracy of <0.5 mm reported by Diaz et al. [DKG+13], where the laser ablation was exactly guided according to the ablation depth measured with OCT.

Reviewing the candidate sensor technologies introduced in section 2.3.2, the only reasonable choices are the control concepts based on monitoring the laser ablation induced emissions. Preliminary experiments revealed that the ablation plume is unstable while cooling water spray (refer to section 2.2.2) is applied. Therefore, the approach proposed by Ruppert et al. [RTK+03, RTGW+04] which monitors the intensity of the ablation plume is not feasible for our case, either. Consequently, the only remaining candidate is monitoring the acoustic emissions during the ablation process.

Considering that the acoustic emission based approaches can detect the transition from the hard tissue to the underlying soft tissue only after the first pulse applied to the soft tissue layer, a precondition has to be satisfied: the underlying soft tissue has to be thick enough (e.g. dura mater) so that a single laser pulse applied to it will not lead to severe injury to the structure. For the situations satisfying this precondition, a hybrid control concept is conceived as following:

- Phase I:
  The laser ablation is performed as usual and the ablation depth is monitored by the OCT, until a pre-defined "switching" depth is reached.
- Phase II:
  The control module is switched to the acoustic monitoring. Meanwhile, the laser ablation is performed with reduced pulse duration and reduced energy, so that the injury due to the first pulses applied to the underlying soft tissue can be kept to a minimal level. As soon as a tissue transition is detected, the laser ablation will be terminated.

Having discovered that the conventional Fourier transform based methods are not robust enough for monitoring single laser pulses with reduced energy, wavelet analysis is chosen as the mathematical tool to distinguish pulses applied on hard and soft tissues. Preliminary experiments proved the feasibility of this new approach. Thus, the acoustic emission based tissue boundary detection would be a promising candidate to supplement the OCT for the case of narrow incisions and to terminate the ablation as soon as the first pulse is applied to the underlying soft tissue layer. A closed-loop control of the laser bone ablation with limited injury to the underlying soft tissue could be developed based on this concept in the future, which may provide an "ear" to the OCT guided laser ablation system.

Bibliography

[AB07] Oliver F Adunka and Craig A Buchman. Scala tympani cochleostomy i: results of a survey. *The Laryngoscope*, 117(12):2187–2194, 2007.

[AF59] Antonio Ascenzi and Claudine Fabry. Technique for dissection and measurement of refractive index of osteones. *The Journal of biophysical and biochemical cytology*, 6(1): 139–142, 1959.

[AGAL10] Mirko Arnold, Anarta Ghosh, Stefan Ameling, and Gerard Lacey. Automatic segmentation and inpainting of specular highlights for endoscopic imaging. *Journal on Image and Video Processing*, 2010:9, 2010.

[AJ63] L Allen and DGC Jones. An analysis of the granularity of scattered optical maser light. *Physics Letters*, 7(5):321–323, 1963.

[AKF04] Desmond C Adler, Tony H Ko, and James G Fujimoto. Speckle reduction in optical coherence tomography images by use of a spatially adaptive wavelet filter. *Optics letters*, 29(24):2878–2880, 2004.

[ARG+07] Oliver F Adunka, Andreas Radeloff, Wolfgang K Gstoettner, Harold C Pillsbury, and Craig A Buchman. Scala tympani cochleostomy ii: topography and histology. *The Laryngoscope*, 117(12):2195–2200, 2007.

[ARG08] ARGES GmbH. *InScript Manual*, 2008.

[ARG13] ARGES GmbH. *Manual: Scan Head version all*, v7.0 edition, 2013.

[BAB10] Gregory J Basura, Oliver F Adunka, and Craig A Buchman. Scala tympani cochleostomy for cochlear implantation. *Operative Techniques in Otolaryngology-Head and Neck Surgery*, 21(4):218–222, 2010.

[Bal81] Dana H Ballard. Generalizing the hough transform to detect arbitrary shapes. *Pattern recognition*, 13(2):111–122, 1981.

[BDZA+14] Peter Brett, Xinli Du, Masoud Zoka-Assadi, Chris Coulson, Andrew Reid, and David Proops. Feasibility study of a hand guided robotic drill for cochleostomy. *BioMed Research International*, 2014.

[BKRW09] Jessica Burgner, Lüder A. Kahrs, Jörg Raczkowsky, and Heinz Wörn. Including parameterization of the discrete ablation process into a planning and simulation environment for robot-assisted laser osteotomy. In *Medicine meets virtual reality*, volume 17, pages 43–48, 2009.

[BLW87] Rolf Bertolini, Gerald Leutert, and Klaus Welt. *Systematische Anatomie des Menschen.* VEB Verlag Volk und Gesundheit, 1987.

[BMRW09] Jessica Burgner, Meiko Mueller, Joerg Raczkowsky, and Heinz Woern. Robot assisted laser bone processing: Marking and cutting experiments. In *Advanced Robotics, 2009. ICAR 2009. International Conference on*, pages 1–6. IEEE, 2009.

[BMRW10] J Burgner, M Müller, J Raczkowsky, and H Wörn. Ex vivo accuracy evaluation for robot assisted laser bone ablation. *The International Journal of Medical Robotics and Computer Assisted Surgery*, 6(4):489–500, 2010.

[BP94] Wolfgang Böhm and Hartmut Prautzsch. *Geometric concepts for geometric design.* Peters, Wellesley, Mass., 1994.

[BR00] M Bashkansky and J Reintjes. Statistics and reduction of speckle in optical coherence tomography. *Optics Letters*, 25(8):545–547, 2000.

[BRW08] J Burgner, J Raczkowsky, and H Wörn. Establishment of an experimental setup for robot assisted laser osteotomy with corresponding simulation environment for optimization of all relevant parameters. *Proceedings of the curac*, 8:147–148, 2008.

[BSV13] Jorge Bernal, Javier Sanchez, and Fernando Vilarino. Impact of image preprocessing methods on polyp localization in colonoscopy frames. In *Engineering in Medicine and Biology Society (EMBC), 2013 35th Annual International Conference of the IEEE*, pages 7350–7354, 2013.

[BTSR05] Robert JS Briggs, Michael Tykocinski, Katrina Stidham, and Joseph B Roberson. Cochleostomy site: implications for electrode placement and hearing preservation. *Acta oto-laryngologica*, 125(8):870–876, 2005.

[Bur10] Jessica Burgner. *Robot assisted laser osteotomy.* PhD thesis, Karlsruhe Institute of Technology, Karlsruhe, 2010.

[CC07] Ming-Fei Chen and Yu-Pin Chen. Compensating technique of field-distorting error for the co_2 laser galvanometric scanning drilling machines. *International Journal of Machine Tools and Manufacture*, 47(7):1114–1124, 2007.

[CCA92] Isaac Cohen, Laurent D Cohen, and Nicholas Ayache. Using deformable surfaces to segment 3-d images and infer differential structures. *CVGIP: Image understanding*, 56(2):242–263, 1992.

[CCH09] Ming-Fei Chen, Yu-Pin Chen, and Wen-Tse Hsiao. Correction of field distortion of laser marking systems using surface compensation function. *Optics and Lasers in Engineering*, 47(1):84–89, 2009.

[CET98] Timothy F Cootes, Gareth J Edwards, and Christopher J Taylor. Active appearance models. In *Computer Vision–ECCV'98*, pages 484–498. Springer, 1998.

[CFF09] Shahab Chitchian, Michael A Fiddy, and Nathaniel M Fried. Denoising during optical coherence tomography of the prostate nerves via wavelet shrinkage using dual-tree complex wavelet transform. *Journal of biomedical optics*, 14(1):014031–014031, 2009.

[CJEDS+98] Bill W Colston Jr, Matthew J Everett, Luiz B Da Silva, Linda L Otis, Pieter Stroeve, Howard Nathel, et al. Imaging of hard-and soft-tissue structure in the oral cavity by optical coherence tomography. *Applied Optics*, 37(16):3582–3585, 1998.

[CK72] CK Chow and T Kaneko. Automatic boundary detection of the left ventricle from cineangiograms. *Computers and biomedical research*, 5(4):388–410, 1972.

[CLT+07] Yu Cao, Danyu Liu, Wallapak Tavanapong, Johnny Wong, Jung Hwan Oh, and Piet C de Groen. Computer-aided detection of diagnostic and therapeutic operations in colonoscopy videos. *Biomedical Engineering, IEEE Transactions on*, 54(7):1268–1279, 2007.

[Coh97] Noel L Cohen. Cochlear implant soft surgery: Fact or fantasy? *Otolaryngology-Head and Neck Surgery*, 117(3): 214–216, 1997.

[CPW90] Wai-Fung Cheong, Scott A Prahl, and Ashley J Welch. A review of the optical properties of biological tissues. *Quantum Electronics, IEEE Journal of*, 26(12):2166–2185, 1990.

[CSYI03] Michael A Choma, Marinko V Sarunic, Changhuei Yang, and Joseph A Izatt. Sensitivity advantage of swept source and fourier domain optical coherence tomography. *Optics Express*, 11(18):2183–2189, 2003.

[CT92] Timothy F Cootes and Christopher J Taylor. Active shape models–'smart snakes'. In *BMVC92*, pages 266–275. Springer, 1992.

[CTCG95] Timothy F Cootes, Christopher J Taylor, David H Cooper, and Jim Graham. Active shape models-their training and application. *Computer vision and image understanding*, 61(1):38–59, 1995.

[CYV00] S Grace Chang, Bin Yu, and Martin Vetterli. Spatially adaptive wavelet thresholding with context modeling for image denoising. *Image Processing, IEEE Transactions on*, 9(9):1522–1531, 2000.

[CZWX09] Suochao Cui, Xiao Zhu, Wei Wang, and Yunhui Xie. Calibration of a laser galvanometric scanning system by adapting a camera model. *Applied optics*, 48(14):2632–2637, 2009.

[DAJ+13] Xinli Du, Masoud Z Assadi, Felicity Jowitt, Peter N Brett, Scott Henshaw, James Dalton, David W Proops, Chris J Coulson, and Andrew P Reid. Robustness analysis of a smart surgical drill for cochleostomy. *The International Journal of Medical Robotics and Computer Assisted Surgery*, 9(1):119–126, 2013.

[DBCP+03] Johannes F De Boer, Barry Cense, B Hyle Park, Mark C Pierce, Guillermo J Tearney, and Brett E Bouma. Improved signal-to-noise ratio in spectral-domain compared with time-domain optical coherence tomography. *Optics letters*, 28(21):2067–2069, 2003.

[DF08] W. Drexler and J. G. Fujimoto. *Optical coherence tomography: technology and applications.* Springer, 2008.

[Dij59] Edsger W Dijkstra. A note on two problems in connexion with graphs. *Numerische mathematik*, 1(1):269–271, 1959.

[DiM12] Charles A. DiMarzio. *Optics for engineers.* CRC Press, Boca Raton, Fla. [u.a.], 2012.

[dJBB+13] Sam Van der Jeught, Jan A N Buytaert, Adrian Bradu, Adrian Gh Podoleanu, and Joris J J Dirckx. Real-time correction of geometric distortion artefacts in large-volume optical coherence tomography. *Measurement Science and Technology*, 24(5):057001, 2013.

[DKG+13] Jesús Díaz Díaz, Dennis Kundrat, Kim-Fat Goh, Omid Majdani, and Tobias Ortmaier. Towards intra-operative oct guidance for automatic head surgery: First experimental results. In *Medical Image Computing and Computer-Assisted Intervention–MICCAI 2013*, pages 347–354. Springer, 2013.

[DS98] Nicolae Duta and Milan Sonka. Segmentation and interpretation of mr brain images. an improved active shape model. *Medical Imaging, IEEE Transactions on*, 17(6):1049–1062, 1998.

[DVO+07] AE Desjardins, BJ Vakoc, WY Oh, SMR Motaghiannezam, GJ Tearney, and BE Bouma. Angle-resolved optical coherence tomography with sequential angular selectivity for speckle reduction. *Optics express*, 15(10):6200, 2007.

[DYQS04] Ye Duan, Liu Yang, Hong Qin, and Dimitris Samaras. Shape reconstruction from 3d and 2d data using pde-based deformable surfaces. In *Computer Vision-ECCV 2004*, pages 238–251. Springer, 2004.

[EBO+09] H. Eilers, S. Baron, T. Ortmaier, B. Heimann, C. Baier, T.S. Rau, M. Leinung, and O. Majdani. Navigated, robot assisted drilling of a minimally invasive cochlear access. In *Mechatronics, 2009. ICM 2009. IEEE International Conference on*, pages 1–6, April 2009.

[EE06] Jürgen Eichler and Hans Joachim Eichler. *Laser: Bauformen, Strahlführung, Anwendung.* Springer, 2006.

[EWO+09] H Eilers, M Wienke, T Ortmaier, O Majdani, and M Leinung. Surgical navigation. *Int J CARS*, 4(1):S124–S133, 2009.

[FKS+12] A Fuchs, D Kundrat, M Schultz, A Krüger, and T Ortmaier. Automatisierte überwachung der laserosteotomie mittels optischer kohärenztomographie. *Tagungsband der 11. Jahrestagung der Deutschen Gesellschaft für Computer- und Roboterassistierte Chirurgie e.V.*, 2012.

[FLN+12] Leyuan Fang, Shutao Li, Qing Nie, Joseph A. Izatt, Cynthia A. Toth, and Sina Farsiu. Sparsity based denoising of spectral domain optical coherence tomography images. *Biomed. Opt. Express*, 3(5):927–942, May 2012.

[FS00] J.M. Fitzpatrick and M. Sonka. *Handbook of Medical Imaging: Medical Image Processing and Analysis.* Handbook of Medical Imaging. SPIE Press, 2000.

[FSK+12] A Fuchs, M Schultz, A Krüger, D Kundrat, J Díaz Díaz, and T Ortmaier. Online measurement and evaluation of the er: Yag laser ablation process using an integrated oct system. *Biomed Tech*, 57:1, 2012.

[Fuj01] James G Fujimoto. Optical coherence tomography. *Comptes Rendus de l'Académie des Sciences-Series IV-Physics*, 2(8):1099–1111, 2001.

[Fuj06] Jim Fujimoto. Optical coherence tomography. In *Conference on Lasers and Electro-Optics*. Optical Society of America, 2006.

[GSEM11] Michaël JA Girard, Nicholas G Strouthidis, C Ross Ethier, and Jean Martial Mari. Shadow removal and contrast enhancement in optical coherence tomography images of the human optic nerve head. *Investigative Ophthalmology & Visual Science*, 52(10):7738–7748, 2011.

[GSV12] Anne M. [Hrsg.] Gilroy, Michael Schünke, and Markus [Ill.] Voll, editors. *Atlas of anatomy*. Thieme, Stuttgart, 2nd ed. edition, 2012. Includes index.

[GTFP04] UW Geisthoff, Steffen H Tretbar, Ph A Federspil, and Peter K Plinkert. Improved ultrasound-based navigation for robotic drilling at the lateral skull base. In *International Congress Series*, volume 1268, pages 662–666. Elsevier, 2004.

[GW02] Rafael C. Gonzalez and Richard E. Woods. *Digital image processing*. Prentice-Hall, Upper Saddle River, NJ, 2. ed. edition, 2002.

[GW14] Mona K Garvin and Xiaodong Wu. Graph algorithmic techniques for biomedical image segmentation. In *Advanced Computational Approaches to Biomedical Engineering*, pages 3–45. Springer, 2014.

[HD97] David I Hughes and Francis A Duck. Automatic attenuation compensation for ultrasonic imaging. *Ultrasound in medicine & biology*, 23(5):651–664, 1997.

[HFI+08] Matthias B Hullin, Martin Fuchs, Ivo Ihrke, Hans-Peter Seidel, and Hendrik Lensch. Fluorescent immersion range scanning. In *ACM Transactions on Graphics (TOG)*, volume 27, page 87. ACM, 2008.

[Hou62] Paul VC Hough. Method and means for recognizing complex patterns, December 18 1962. US Patent 3,069,654.

[HSL+91] David Huang, Eric A Swanson, Charles P Lin, Joel S Schuman, William G Stinson, Warren Chang, Michael R Hee, Thomas Flotte, Kenton Gregory, Carmen A Puliafito, et al. Optical coherence tomography. *Science*, 254(5035):1178–1181, 1991.

[HWA+07] Mona Haeker, Xiaodong Wu, Michael Abràmoff, Randy Kardon, and Milan Sonka. Incorporation of regional information in optimal 3-d graph search with application for intraretinal layer segmentation of optical coherence tomography images. In *Information Processing in Medical Imaging*, pages 607–618. Springer, 2007.

[HWF06] R Huber, M Wojtkowski, and JG Fujimoto. Fourier domain mode locking (fdml): A new laser operating regime and applications for optical coherence tomography. *Optics Express*, 14(8):3225–3237, 2006.

[HZ02] Eugene Hecht and Alfred Zajac. Optics. *Addison-Wesley*, 2:163–169, 2002.

[IBT03] Nicusor Iftimia, Brett E Bouma, and Guillermo J Tearney. Speckle reduction in optical coherence tomography by "path length encoded" angular compounding. *Journal of biomedical optics*, 8(2):260–263, 2003.

[IH98] Mikhail Ivanenko and Peter Hering. Wet bone ablation with mechanically Q-switched high-repetion-rate CO_2 laser. *Applied Physics B: Lasers and Optics*, Bd. 67(3):395–397, 1998.

[IKY+97] Joseph A Izatt, Manish D Kulkarni, Siavash Yazdanfar, Jennifer K Barton, and Ashley J Welch. In vivo bidirectional color doppler flow imaging of picoliter blood volumes using optical coherence tomography. *Optics letters*, 22(18):1439–1441, 1997.

[IWA+05] Mikhail Ivanenko, Martin Werner, Said Afilal, Manfred Klasing, and Peter Hering. Ablation of hard bone tissue with pulsed CO_2 lasers. *Medical Laser Application*, 20: 13–23, 2005.

[JAB+05] Chris James, Klaus Albegger, Rolf Battmer, Sandro Burdo, Naima Deggouj, Olivier Deguine, Norbert Dillier, Michel Gersdorff, Roland Laszig, Thomas Lenarz, et al. Preservation of residual hearing with cochlear implantation: how and why. *Acta oto-laryngologica*, 125(5):481–491, 2005.

[JSS01] Anthony F Jahn and Joseph Santos-Sacchi. *Physiology of the Ear*. Cengage Learning, 2001.

[Kah09] Lüder Alexander Kahrs. *Bildverarbeitungsunterstützte Laserknochenablation am humanen Felsenbein*. PhD thesis, Karlsruher Institut für Technologie, Karlsruhe, 2009.

[KBK+10] Lüder Alexander Kahrs, Jessica Burgner, Thomas Klenzner, Jörg Raczkowsky, Jörg Schipper, and Heinz Wörn. Planning and simulation of microsurgical laser bone ablation. *International journal of computer assisted radiology and surgery*, 5(2):155–162, 2010.

[KCH+11] Brendan F Kennedy, Andrea Curatolo, Timothy R Hillman, Christobel M Saunders, and David D Sampson. Speckle reduction in optical coherence tomography images using tissue viscoelasticity. *Journal of Biomedical Optics*, 16(2):020506–020506, 2011.

[KHCS10] Brendan F Kennedy, Timothy R Hillman, Andrea Curatolo, and David D Sampson. Speckle reduction in optical coherence tomography by strain compounding. *Optics letters*, 35(14):2445–2447, 2010.

[KKS+09] Thomas Klenzner, Felix B Knapp, Joerg Schipper, Joerg Raczkowsky, Heinz Woern, Lueder A Kahrs, Martin Werner, and Peter Hering. High precision cochleostomy by use of a pulsed CO_2 laser–an experimental approach. *Cochlear implants international*, 10(S1):58–62, 2009.

[KNK+09] Thomas Klenzner, ChiuChun Ngan, FelixBernhard Knapp, Hayo Knoop, Jan Kromeier, Antje Aschendorff, Evangelos Papastathopoulos, Joerg Raczkowsky, Heinz Wörn, and Joerg Schipper. New strategies for high precision surgery of the temporal bone using a robotic approach for cochlear implantation. *European Archives of Oto-Rhino-Laryngology*, 266(7):955–960, 2009.

[Kok04] Anil C Kokaram. On missing data treatment for degraded video and film archives: a survey and a new bayesian approach. *Image Processing, IEEE Transactions on*, 13(3):397–415, 2004.

[KOW08] HW Kang, J Oh, and AJ Welch. Investigations on laser hard tissue ablation under various environments. *Physics in medicine and biology*, 53(12):3381, 2008.

[KRW+08] Lüder A Kahrs, Jörg Raczkowsky, Martin Werner, Felix B Knapp, Markus Mehrwald, Peter Hering, Jörg Schipper, Thomas Klenzner, and Heinz Wörn. Visual servoing of a laser ablation based cochleostomy. In *Medical imaging*, pages 69182C–69182C. International Society for Optics and Photonics, 2008.

[KWA+12] Thomas Klein, Wolfgang Wieser, Raphael André, Tom Pfeiffer, Christoph M Eigenwillig, and Robert Huber. Multi-mhz fdml oct: snapshot retinal imaging at 6.7 million axial-scans per second. In *SPIE BiOS*, pages 82131E–82131E. International Society for Optics and Photonics, 2012.

[KWK+07] LA Kahrs, M Werner, FB Knapp, S-F Lu, J Raczkowsky, J Schipper, M Ivanenko, H Wörn, P Hering, and Th Klenzner. Video camera based navigation of a laser beam for micro surgery bone ablation at the skull base-setup and initial experiments. In *Advances in Medical Engineering*, pages 219–223. Springer, 2007.

[KWT88] Michael Kass, Andrew Witkin, and Demetri Terzopoulos. Snakes: Active contour models. *International journal of computer vision*, 1(4):321–331, 1988.

[LCG+08] R Lapeer, MS Chen, G Gonzalez, A Linney, and G Alusi. Image-enhanced surgical navigation for endoscopic sinus surgery: evaluating calibration, registration and tracking. *The International Journal of Medical Robotics and Computer Assisted Surgery*, 4(1):32–45, 2008.

[Leh93] E Lehnhardt. Intracochlear placement of cochlear implant electrodes in soft surgery technique. *HNO*, 41(7):356–359, 1993.

[Leu05] R Leuwer. Gestörtes Hören - die apparative Versorgung der Schwerhörigkeit: Konventionelle und Implantierbare Hörgeräte. *Laryngo-Rhino-Otologie*, 84(S 1):51–61, 2005.

[LFG99] K. Lenfert, T. Fröhlich, and M. Geiger. Gewebeserkennung bei der laserosteotomie in der mkg-chirurgie. In *1. Symposium: Neue Technologien für die Medizin Forschung - Praxis - Innovation*. Herbert Utz Verlag, 1999.

[LHF+03] R Leitgeb, CK Hitzenberger, Adolf F Fercher, et al. Performance of fourier domain vs. time domain optical coherence tomography. *Opt. Express*, 11(8):889–894, 2003.

[LHLS07] M. Leinung, D. Hagner, Th. Lenarz, and B. Schwab. Akustische analyse zur grenzflächedetektion bei der er:yag-cochleostomie. *Tagungsband der 6. Jahrestagung der Deutschen Gesellschaft für Computer- und Roboterassistierte Chirurgie e.V.*, pages 65–68, 2007.

[LIS+09] Irina V Larina, Steven Ivers, Saba Syed, Mary E Dickinson, and Kirill V Larin. Hemodynamic measurements from individual blood cells in early mammalian embryos with doppler swept source oct. *Optics letters*, 34(7):986–988, 2009.

[Liu05] Mingcai Liu. *Wavelet Analysis and Applications*. Tsinghua University Press, Beijing, 2005.

[LWFY12] Ben YC Leung, Paul JL Webster, James M Fraser, and Victor XD Yang. Real-time guidance of thermal and ultrashort pulsed laser ablation in hard tissue using inline coherent imaging. *Lasers in surgery and medicine*, 44(3):249–256, 2012.

[MED09] MED-EL Medical Electronics. http://www.medel.com, Oct. 2009.

[MHTG+11] Frode Manstad-Hulaas, Geir Arne Tangen, Lucian Gheorghe Gruionu, Petter Aadahl, and Toril AN Hernes. Three-dimensional endovascular navigation with electromagnetic tracking: ex vivo and in vivo accuracy. *Journal of Endovascular Therapy*, 18(2):230–240, 2011.

[MMF+08] Maziar Mir, Joerg Meister, Rene Franzen, Shabnam S Sabounchi, Friedrich Lampert, and Norbert Gutknecht. Influence of water-layer thickness on Er:YAG laser ablation of enamel of bovine anterior teeth. *Lasers in medical science*, 23(4):451–457, 2008.

[MRB+09] Omid Majdani, ThomasS. Rau, Stephan Baron, Hubertus Eilers, Claas Baier, Bodo Heimann, Tobias Ortmaier, Sönke Bartling, Thomas Lenarz, and Martin Leinung. A robot-guided minimally invasive approach for cochlear implant surgery: preliminary results of a temporal bone study. *International Journal of Computer Assisted Radiology and Surgery*, 4(5):475–486, 2009.

[MSI11] Alkhazur Manakov, Hans-Peter Seidel, and Ivo Ihrke. A Mathematical Model and Calibration Procedure for Galvanometric Laser Scanning Systems. In *Proceedings of VMV*, pages 207–214, 2011.

[MSRW10] Holger Mönnich, Daniel Stein, Jörg Raczkowsky, and Heinz Wörn. Results of co_2 robotic laser oseotomy in surgery with motion compensation. In *BiOS*, pages 75484A–75484A. International Society for Optics and Photonics, 2010.

[MT99] T McInemey and Demetri Terzopoulos. Topology adaptive deformable surfaces for medical image volume segmentation. *Medical Imaging, IEEE Transactions on*, 18(10): 840–850, 1999.

[MYY09a] Shuichi Makita, Masahiro Yamanari, and Yoshiaki Yasuno. In vivo depth-resolved tissue contrast by local birefringence and differential optic axis orientation using polarization-sensitive swept-source optical coherence tomography. In *Proc. SPIE*, volume 7168, page 71682H, 2009.

[MYY+09b] Zhuo Meng, X Steve Yao, Hui Yao, Yan Liang, Tiegen Liu, Yanni Li, Guanhua Wang, and Shoufeng Lan. Measurement of the refractive index of human teeth by optical coherence tomography. *Journal of biomedical optics*, 14(3):034010–034010, 2009.

[Nga06] Chiu-Chun Ngan. *Atraumatic and function-preserving high precision surgery of the human temporal bone.* Der Andere Verlag, 2006.

[Nie07] Markolf H. Niemz. *Laser-Tissue Interactions: Fundamentals and Applications.* Springer, third, enlarged edition, 2007.

[Nip09] John K Niparko. *Cochlear implants: Principles and practices.* Wolters Kluwer Health, 2009.

[OBD+07] Aydogan Ozcan, Alberto Bilenca, Adrien E Desjardins, Brett E Bouma, and Guillermo J Tearney. Speckle reduction in optical coherence tomography images using digital filtering. *JOSA A*, 24(7):1901–1910, 2007.

[OHL+07] JungHwan Oh, Sae Hwang, JeongKyu Lee, Wallapak Tavanapong, Johnny Wong, and Piet C de Groen. Informative frame classification for endoscopy video. *Medical Image Analysis*, 11(2):110–127, 2007.

[OOYH00] M. Ohmi, Y. Ohnishi, K. Yoden, and M. Haruna. In vitro simultaneous measurement of refractive index and thickness of biological tissue by the low coherence interferometry. *Biomedical Engineering, IEEE Transactions on*, 47(9):1266–1270, 2000.

[OSG+10] Sergio Ortiz, Damian Siedlecki, Ireneusz Grulkowski, Laura Remon, Daniel Pascual, Maciej Wojtkowski, and Susana Marcos. Optical distortion correction in optical coherence tomography for quantitative ocular anterior segment by three-dimensional imaging. *Opt. Express*, 18(3):2782–2796, Feb 2010.

[OSRM09] Sergio Ortiz, Damian Siedlecki, Laura Remon, and Susana Marcos. Optical coherence tomography for quantitative surface topography. *Applied optics*, 48(35):6708–6715, 2009.

[OTFH04] Masato Ohmi, Manabu Tanizawa, Atsushi Fukunaga, and Masamitsu Haruna. Automatic in-situ observation of tissue laser ablation using optical coherence tomography. In *Biophotonics, 2004. APBP 2004. The Second Asian and Pacific Rim Symposium on*, pages 228–229. IEEE, 2004.

[Ots79] Nobuyuki Otsu. A threshold selection method from gray-level histograms. *Systems, Man and Cybernetics, IEEE Transactions on*, 9(1):62–66, 1979.

[PAF+01] Dale Purves, George J Augustine, David Fitzpatrick, Lawrence C Katz, Anthony-Samuel LaMantia, James O McNamara, S Mark Williams, et al. *Neuroscience*, chapter 13. Sinauer Associates, 2nd edition, 2001.

[PB09] Prabakar Puvanathasan and Kostadinka Bizheva. Interval type-ii fuzzy anisotropic diffusion algorithm for speckle noise reduction in optical coherence tomography images. *Optics express*, 17(2):733–746, 2009.

[PBP02] Hartmut Prautzsch, Wolfgang Böhm, and Marco Paluszny. *Bézier and B-spline techniques*. Mathematics + visualization. Springer, Berlin [u.a.], 2002.

[PGL+03] Michael Pircher, Erich Go, Rainer Leitgeb, Adolf F Fercher, Christoph K Hitzenberger, et al. Speckle reduction in optical coherence tomography by frequency compounding. *Journal of Biomedical Optics*, 8(3):565–569, 2003.

[Phy03] Physik Instrumente (PI) GmbH & Co. KG. *Technical Documentation: MS 54E User Manual, M-850 and M-840 Hexapod 6-Axis Positioning Systems, Release 3.6.0*, 17.11.2003.

[PLQS03] PingTan, S. Lin, Long Quan, and Heung-Yeung Shum. Highlight removal by illumination-constrained inpainting. In *Computer Vision, 2003. Proceedings. Ninth IEEE International Conference on*, pages 164–169 vol.1, 2003.

[PPBS96] F. Pedrotti, L. Pedrotti, Werner Bausch, and Hartmut Schmidt. *Optik: eine Einführung*. Prentice Hall, 1996.

[RBB03] Jadwiga Rogowska, Clifford M Bryant, and Mark E Brezinski. Image processing technique for semiautomatic detection of cartilage boundaries on oct images. In *Lasers and Electro-Optics, 2003. CLEO'03. Conference on*, pages 2–pp. IEEE, 2003.

[RG97] JD Rigden and EI Gordon. The granularity of scattered optical maser light. *SPIE MILESTONE SERIES MS*, 133:213–213, 1997.

[RPS+08] Jörg Ruppin, Aleksandra Popovic, Mario Strauss, Elmar Spüntrup, Alexander Steiner, and Christian Stoll. Evaluation of the accuracy of three different computer-aided surgery systems in dental implantology: optical tracking vs. stereolithographic splint systems. *Clinical oral implants research*, 19(7):709–716, 2008.

[RRL95] M Rogowski, G Reiss, and E Lehnhardt. Morphologic study of the guinea pig cochlea after cochlear implantation using the" soft surgery" technique. *The Annals of otology, rhinology & laryngology. Supplement*, 166:434, 1995.

[RSKW+04] A. Rätzer-Scheibe, M. Klasing, M. Werner, M. Ivanenko, and P. Hering. Acoustic monitoring of bone ablation using pulsed CO_2-lasers. *Aktuelle Methoden der Laser- und Medizinphysik*, pages 281–286, 2004.

[RTGW+04] Stephan Rupprecht, Katja Tangermann-Gerk, Joerg Wiltfang, Friedrich Wilhelm Neukam, and Andreas Schlegel. Sensor-based laser ablation for tissue specific cutting: an experimental study. *Lasers in medical science*, 19(2):81–88, 2004.

[RTK+03] Stephan Rupprecht, Katja Tangermann, Peter Kessler, Friedrich Wilhelm Neukam, and Joerg Wiltfang. Er: Yag laser osteotomy directed by sensor controlled systems. *Journal of Cranio-Maxillofacial Surgery*, 31(6): 337–342, 2003.

[RW06] Peter S Rolanda and Charles G Wrighta. Surgical aspects of cochlear implantation: Mechanisms of insertional trauma. *Cochlear and Brainstem Implants*, 64:11–30, 2006.

[SCA06] SCANLAB AG. *Installation and Operation: The RTC® 4 PC Interface Board for Real Time Control of Scan Heads and Lasers*, rev. 1.3 e edition, 2006.

[Sch97] JM Schmitt. Array detection for speckle reduction in optical coherence microscopy. *Physics in Medicine and Biology*, 42(7):1427, 1997.

[Sch99] Joseph M Schmitt. Optical coherence tomography (OCT): a review. *Selected Topics in Quantum Electronics, IEEE Journal of*, 5(4):1205–1215, 1999.

[Sch07] Dieter Schuöcker. *Spanlose Fertigung*. Oldenbourg Verlag München Wien, 2007.

[SKB93] JM Schmitt, A Knüttel, and RF Bonner. Measurement of optical properties of biological tissues by low-coherence reflectometry. *Applied Optics*, 32(30):6032–6042, 1993.

[SW10] Volker Schulze and Patricia Weber. Precise ablation milling with ultrashort pulsed Nd:YAG lasers by optical and acoustical process control. In *LASE*, pages 75850J–75850J. International Society for Optics and Photonics, 2010.

[SWK+07] H. Steigerwald, M. Werner, M. Klasing, M. Ivanenko, D. Harbechke, C. Wagner, and P. Hering. Spectral analysis of the acoustic signal during ablation of biological tissue with pulsed CO_2-lasers. *Advance in Medical Engineering*, pages 425–430, 2007.

[SXY99] Joseph M Schmitt, SH Xiang, and Kin M Yung. Speckle in optical coherence tomography. *Journal of Biomedical Optics*, 4(1):95–105, 1999.

[TDP+10] R Taylor, X Du, D Proops, A Reid, C Coulson, and P N Brett. A sensory-guided surgical micro-drill. *Proceedings of the Institution of Mechanical Engineers, Part C: Journal of Mechanical Engineering Science*, 224(7):1531–1537, 2010.

[Ter80] Demetri Terzopoulos. On matching deformable models to images. In *Optical Society of America, Topical Meeting on Machine Vision*, volume 1, pages 160–163, 1980.

[TF88] Demetri Terzopoulos and Kurt Fleischer. Deformable models. *The Visual Computer*, 4(6):306–331, 1988.

[TFMY12] Johannes Totz, Kenko Fujii, Peter Mountney, and Guang-Zhong Yang. Enhanced visualisation for minimally invasive surgery. *International Journal of Computer Assisted Radiology and Surgery*, 7(3):423–432, 2012.

[THST95] H Takahashi, I Honjo, I Sando, and A Takagi. Orientation for cochlear implant surgery in cases with round window obstruction: a computer reconstruction study. *European archives of oto-rhino-laryngology*, 252(2):102–105, 1995.

[TPF09] Steffen H Tretbar, Peter K Plinkert, and Philipp A Federspil. Accuracy of ultrasound measurements for skull bone thickness using coded signals. *Biomedical Engineering, IEEE Transactions on*, 56(3):733–740, 2009.

[Tre10] Marco Treiber. *An Introduction to Object Recognition: Selected Algorithms for a Wide Variety of Applications.* Springer, 2010.

[UMA04] Nadya Ugryumova, Stephen John Matcher, and Don P Attenburrow. Measurement of bone mineral density via light scattering. *Physics in medicine and biology*, 49(3):469, 2004.

[vJZZG13] Christopher R von Jako, Yuval Zuk, Oded Zur, and Pini Gilboa. A novel accurate minioptical tracking system for percutaneous needle placement. *Biomedical Engineering, IEEE Transactions on*, 60(8):2222–2225, 2013.

[VPH+02] Florian Vogt, Dietrich Paulus, Benno Heigl, Christian Vogelgsang, Heinrich Niemann, Gunther Greiner, and Christoph Schick. Making the invisible visible: highlight substitution by color light fields. In *Conference on Colour in Graphics, Imaging, and Vision*, volume 2002, pages 352–357. Society for Imaging Science and Technology, 2002.

[VV03] Alfred Vogel and Vasan Venugopalan. Mechanisms of Pulsed Laser Ablation of Biological Tissues. *Chemical Review*, 2003.

[WBK+10] Wolfgang Wieser, Benjamin R Biedermann, Thomas Klein, Christoph M Eigenwillig, and Robert Huber. Multimegahertz oct: High quality 3d imaging at 20 million a-scans and 4.5 gvoxels per second. *Optics express*, 18(14):14685–14704, 2010.

[WD08] Blake S Wilson and Michael F Dorman. Cochlear implants: current designs and future possibilities. *J Rehabil Res Dev*, 45(5):695–730, 2008.

[Wer06] Martin Werner. *Ablation of hard biological tissue and osteotomy with pulsed CO_2 lasers.* PhD thesis, University Düsseldorf, 2006.

[WLS+13] Donglin Wang, Peng Liang, Sean Samuelson, Hongzhi Jia, Junshan Ma, and Huikai Xie. Correction of image distortions in endoscopic optical coherence tomography based on two-axis scanning mems mirrors. *Biomed. Opt. Express*, 4(10):2066–2077, Oct 2013.

[WMBC10] Alexander Wong, Akshaya Mishra, Kostadinka Bizheva, and David A Clausi. General bayesian estimation for speckle noise reduction in optical coherence tomography retinal imagery. *Opt. Express*, 18(8):8338–8352, 2010.

[WPE+12] Wolfgang Wieser, Gesa Palte, Christoph M Eigenwillig, Benjamin R Biedermann, Tom Pfeiffer, and Robert Huber. Chromatic polarization effects of swept waveforms in fdml lasers and fiber spools. *Optics Express*, 20(9):9819–9832, 2012.

[WR09] Hui Wang and Andrew M Rollins. Speckle reduction in optical coherence tomography using angular compounding by b-scan doppler-shift encoding. *Journal of biomedical optics*, 14(3):030512–030512, 2009.

[WRRI02] Volker Westphal, Andrew Rollins, Sunita Radhakrishnan, and Joseph Izatt. Correction of geometric and refractive image distortions in optical coherence tomography applying fermat's principle. *Opt. Express*, 10(9):397–404, 2002.

[WSM+01] Peter K Weber, Joerg C Schlegel, Juergen Meiche, Leonora Peter, and Ulrich Harland. A system for ultrasound based intraoperative navigation in spine surgery. In *Ultrasonics Symposium, 2001 IEEE*, volume 2, pages 1361–1364. IEEE, 2001.

[Wu87] TANG Wu. Characteristics of a double galvanometer deflection system with a distortion lens. *Acta Opt. Sin*, 7:261–268, 1987.

[XHD+05] Jun Xie, Shuhuai Huang, Zhengcheng Duan, Yusheng Shi, and Shifeng Wen. Correction of the image distortion for laser galvanometric scanning system. *Optics & Laser Technology*, 37(4):305 – 311, 2005.

[XP97] Chenyang Xu and Jerry L Prince. Gradient vector flow: A new external force for snakes. In *Computer Vision and Pattern Recognition, 1997. Proceedings., 1997 IEEE Computer Society Conference on*, pages 66–71. IEEE, 1997.

[XSD+11] Lei Xu, Branislav Stojkovic, Hu Ding, Qi Song, Xiaodong Wu, Milan Sonka, and Jinhui Xu. Faster segmentation algorithm for optical coherence tomography images with guaranteed smoothness. In Kenji Suzuki, Fei Wang, Dinggang Shen, and Pingkun Yan, editors, *Machine Learning in Medical Imaging*, volume 7009 of *Lecture Notes in Computer Science*, pages 308–316. Springer Berlin Heidelberg, 2011.

[XSD+12] Lei Xu, Branislav Stojkovic, Hu Ding, Qi Song, Xiaodong Wu, Milan Sonka, and Jinhui Xu. Efficient searching of globally optimal and smooth multisurfaces with shape priors. In *SPIE Medical Imaging*, pages 83140N–83140N. International Society for Optics and Photonics, 2012.

[XSZ+11] Lei Xu, Branislav Stojkovic, Yongding Zhu, Qi Song, Xiaodong Wu, Milan Sonka, and Jinhui Xu. Efficient algorithms for segmenting globally optimal and smooth multisurfaces. In *Information Processing in Medical Imaging*, pages 208–220. Springer, 2011.

[YA02] Yongjian Yu and Scott T Acton. Speckle reducing anisotropic diffusion. *Image Processing, IEEE Transactions on*, 11(11):1260–1270, 2002.

[YTdB+03] Seok-Hyun Yun, Guillermo J Tearney, Johannes F de Boer, N Iftimia, and Brett E Bouma. High-speed optical frequency-domain imaging. *Optics Express*, 11(22):2953, 2003.

[YY97] Francis T. S. Yu and Xiangyang Yang. *Introduction to optical engineering*. Cambridge University Press, Cambridge, 1997.

[ZB85] M Zrunek and K Burian. Risk of basilar membrane perforation by intracochlear electrodes. *Archives of oto-rhino-laryngology*, 242(3):295–299, 1985.

[ZFSS00] A V Zvyagin, J B FitzGerald, K Silva, and D D Sampson. Real-time detection technique for doppler optical coherence tomography. *Optics Letters*, 25(22):1645–1647, 2000.

[Zha00] Zhengyou Zhang. A flexible new technique for camera calibration. *Pattern Analysis and Machine Intelligence, IEEE Transactions on*, 22(11):1330–1334, 2000.

[ZJNC04] Jun Zhang, Woonggyu Jung, J Stuart Nelson, and Zhongping Chen. Full range polarization-sensitive fourier domain optical coherence tomography. *Opt. Express*, 12(24):6033–6039, 2004.